A-Z

of *Traditional*
Herbal Remedies

MICHAEL HOWARD

SENATE

A-Z of Traditional Herbal Remedies

First published in 1987 as *Traditional Folk Remedies* by
Century Hutchinson Ltd, London

This edition published in 1997 by Senate,
an imprint of Random House UK Ltd, Random House,
20 Vauxhall Bridge Road, London SW1V 2SA

Copyright © Michael Howard 1987

ISBN 1 85958 504 3

Printed and bound in Guernsey by The Guernsey Press Co Ltd

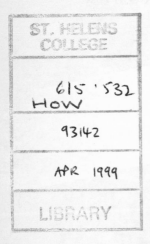

For
LINDA
with love

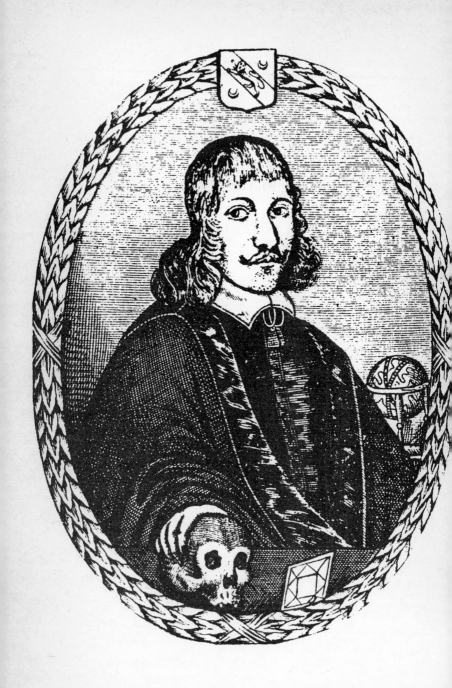

Contents

Acknowledgements

I would like to thank the following who have been of valuable assistance in the preparation of this book; the staff of the Wellcome Institute for the History of Medicine; the staff of the British Library; the staff of Carmarthen Reference Library; the staff of the Westminster Reference Library; the staff of the Folklore Society Library; the staff of University College, London; the staff of the British Museum; Mrs May Griffiths of Carmarthen, Dyfed; Mrs Kathleen Warner of Halstead, Essex; Mr L.A. Marsh of Thorpe Bay, Essex; Mr L. Percival of Devizes, Wiltshire; A.L. Pickering of Holyhead, Anglesey; Mrs L. Sands of Hastings, East Sussex; Hilda Francis of Oswestry, Shropshire; Mrs S. Montgomery of Didcot, Oxfordshire; John Geddes of Stroud, Gloucestershire; Mrs N. Bate of Littleover, Derbyshire; Mrs S.D. Guyatt of Benfleet, Essex; Christine Webber of Cullompton, Devon; Mrs Morfydd Septima-Douse of Devizes, Wiltshire; J. Newcombe of Wellingborough, Northamptonshire; Tom Richards of Bury St Edmunds, Suffolk; Mrs J.G. Brooks of Chester; Miss J. Park-Robertson of Kirkcaldy, Fife; A. Akroyd of Huddersfield, West Yorkshire; J.R. Green of Abingdon, Oxfordshire; C. Hinton of Wanborough, Wiltshire; Mrs P. Lowe of Hillingdon, Greater London; Miss E.K. Caiger of Wallingford, Oxfordshire; Miss P. Patterson of Huddersfield, West Yorkshire; Sonia Lowrey of Trowbridge, Wiltshire; M. Heathorn of Clacton-on-Sea, Essex; Albert Simmonds of Elmswell, Suffolk; R.E. Newton of Rayleigh, Essex; E.J. Parminter of Aylesbury, Buckinghamshire; Hilda Eldred of Newport, Dyfed; and Mrs W. Stoner of Chippenham, Wiltshire.

Michael Howard
West Wales
1986

Part One

A Short History of Folk Healing

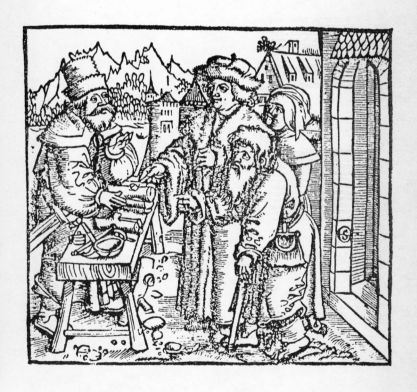

The history of folk medicine dates back many thousands of years; in fact, so closely linked are traditional folk practices and conventional medicine that until comparatively recent times it is difficult to distinguish between them. In the New Stone Age (*c*. 5000 BCE) early mankind was well aware of the medical use of a wide range of healing plants, and in 1963 archaeologists who opened the prehistoric grave of a man buried in a cave near Shedinar in Iraq uncovered evidence of the extent of this ancient knowledge. Scientific analysis of the dust in which the skeletal remains were found revealed that the corpse had been interred surrounded by flowers, which obviously had a religious significance. The flowers were all discovered to have had medicinal properties; the healing plants in this prehistoric grave included diuretics, emetics, astringents, stimulants and pain relievers.

In addition to traditional folk medicine based on healing plants, archaeological remains offer evidence of primitive types of surgery practised in Neolithic times. Saws made of flint, stone and bone have been unearthed from Neolithic burial places, and some skeletal remains dated from this period display signs of trepanning and the amputation of limbs; evidence of circumcision and ritual tattooing has also been found. Bronze Age (*c*. 2000 BCE) surgical saws and other medical tools have been identified by archaeologists examining graves of that period in both Europe and the Middle East. The use of naturally narcotic drugs such as opium, mandrake, hemlock and cocaine was also widespread in ancient cultures for medical purposes, and natural antiseptics such as honey, vinegar, salt and alcohol were commonly employed for cleaning open wounds.

This traditional knowledge of folk remedies survives today among traditional peoples, even when they are uprooted from their ancient homelands. In Brazil folk remedies based on herbal ingredients are still used extensively by the slum dwellers who have moved from the jungle to the outskirts of the cities. Dr Celerio Carriconde, an expert in the various different forms of alternative medicine who has spent many years in Uruguay, Chile, Panama and Brazil researching folk remedies, discovered that in rural areas of Panama honey was widely used as an antiseptic, especially during childbirth. Subsequent scientific research has proved that honey contains a bactericidal agent. It is evident from Dr Carriconde's research work that traditional folk medicine as practised by tribal and post-tribal communities produces results comparable to those obtained from the use of more conventional medical products.

The majority of cures achieved with folk medicine and folk remedies were based on natural extracts from well-known plants which the ancient peoples discovered, by trial and error, had the ability to heal various ailments. Before the invention of writing, knowledge about these plants was passed on orally, accompanied by semi-magical rituals within a religious context. This aura of mystery and magic was often deliberately cultivated by the folk healers in ancient tribal communities; healing and folk medicine became an esoteric art practised by the priest or priestess and regarded as the gift of the gods. As religious consciousness became more sophisticated the healing arts became the specific province of gods and goddesses who ruled over this important aspect of human life; the priesthood who served these deities took the social role of healer and physician within the community by divine right. It was only gradually that this monopoly was breached through the use of simple folk remedies by ordinary people; but despite the spread of knowledge about folk medicine, the *modus operandi* of medical practice retained its atmosphere of religious sanctity, even though in later centuries this degenerated into superstition and half-remembered magical rites.

With the invention of writing, information on herbalism and folk remedies spread to a wider section of the community, although it was still limited to the social élite who could read and write. The first herbals on healing plants are from China, dated *c*. 3000 BCE; the Emperor Shen Nung (2737–2697 BCE) published a medical treatise listing over 260 medical preparations based on herbs, and sixty years later the Emperor Huangh wrote what is now recognized as the first medical treatise listing diseases and their cures. The history of medical herbalism in China is a long one, and by 800 CE it is recorded that Chinese physicians had access to over eleven thousand different prescriptions. Standard medical textbooks were in wide circulation among the healing profession, and a highly organized system of medical practitioners existed.

In India the Hindu sacred book known as the *Rig Veda*, dating from 2000–1500 BCE, contains several references to physicians. At this time they were regarded as an unclean caste and were socially segregated; a possible reason was that their mission as healers brought them into daily contact with the lower levels of Indian society, who were much in need of their expertise. By the second and third centuries BCE medical support establishments similiar to modern hospitals had been set up by Buddhist monks throughout the Indian sub-continent. Chinese travellers in India during this period described them eloquently as 'houses of mercy for the sick', a description which suggests that some may have served as hospices for the terminally ill.

In addition to their herbal wisdom, Buddhist and Hindu physicians could also boast a knowledge of anatomy and surgical procedures which were not even to be achieved by many medieval doctors in Europe. From the ancient Indian medical treatises we know that their physicians divided the supra-orbital nerve for neuralgia, undertook laparotomy for intestinal obstruction and practised suture of the bowels for internal injury. Their knowledge of anatomy seems to have been based on dissection, for which purpose they used the bodies of children under two years of age who had died of natural causes. This age limit was imposed for religious reasons, for by Hindu custom anyone over that age was cremated after death.

It was not only in the ancient Far East that herbalism and folk medicine flourished. In a region of the Middle Eastern country of Mesopotamia which is now part of Syria, the Sumerians had developed sophisticated medical skills. In common with many ancient peoples they believed that disease was the physical manifestation of demonic possession and psychic attack. This is not really so bizarre as it first seems, for modern medical research is slowly proving that many illnesses are related to psychological states of mind and that their physical symptoms are merely a reflection of inner conflicts within the human psyche. The Sumerians believed, however, that these psychically induced complaints would respond to the healing balm of plants which grew prolifically in the area.

The earliest Sumerian medical herbals date from 2500 BCE, but it is possible even older versions exist which have not survived the ravages of time. The Assyrian civilization succeeded that of the Sumerians, in the same region, about a thousand years later. Tablets from the library of Ashurbanipal, King of Assyria between 662 and 626 BCE, reveal that at that period knowledge of herbs with healing abilities was considerable. Over two hundred and fifty natural drugs derived from local plants are described, which suggests that the propagation of medical plants had become a specialized undertaking. The Sumerians also possessed other advanced medical expertise, including surgical skill: they had, for example, some basic idea of urinology (examination of the urine for evidence of infections and diseases); this is shown by the title of one of their physicians – Asu, or 'one who knows water'.

It is difficult to say whether or not a knowledge of herbalism was a natural by-product of civilization in the Middle East, or whether it was imported from outside. In ancient Egypt the first historically recorded physician was Imhotep, allegedly the physician who served the Pharaoh Zoser in the Third Dynasty, c. 2980 BCE. As well as being a court physician, Imhotep was said to have been an astrologer, magician and psychic healer; after his death he was deified and entered the pantheon of Egyptian gods as the patron of medicine.

Several other ancient Egyptian gods and goddesses were also connected with the art of healing. The principal deity of healing was the lion-headed goddess Sekhmet, who in Egyptian mythology represented the creative force of the sun which has healing power. Her powers could, however, be double-edged, for Sekhmet was also credited with causing plagues. By a strange logic, because the goddess was supposed to be the originator of certain diseases it was also within her power to heal those afflicted with these maladies.

Another Egyptian god associated with healing was Set or Seth, the ass-headed brother of Isis and Osiris. His original role seems to have been as a guide to the dead, transporting them to the underworld. He was also the patron of the priests, whose task it was to embalm the dead and perform funeral rites. When Set's followers rebelled against the established priesthood of Isis and Osiris he was transformed into the personification of evil, and his previous divine duties as the helper of the dead were taken over by the jackal-headed god Anubis, son of Isis.

During the days of the Old Kingdom in Egypt the ibis-headed moon god Thoth or Tehuti was recognized as the patron of medicine. This connection lasted into Greco-Roman times, when Thoth's attributes were combined with those of the Greek god of healing, Hermes. According to ancient myth it was Thoth who discovered the medical properties of herbs, and he was said to be the author of the first herbals used by the priesthood.

Medical payri were the closely guarded property of the priesthood, who kept them locked away in the temples which no outsider dared enter. The earliest Egyptian herbal, said to date from 2800 BCE, records various herbs, aromatic gums and spices used for medical purposes; they included frankincense, cinnamon and cassia. It also contains recipes for herbal ointments manufactured by extracting the plant oil from selected herbs or by mixing them with castor oil. It would seem from the available archaeological evidence that around 2000 BCE spices, herbs and aromatics were imported into Egypt in large quantities from southern Arabia and the Far East. During this period the Phoenicians, a seafaring merchant race, regularly transported herbs and spices from the Middle East to barter for salt and tin in Spain and northern Europe.

The so-called Ebers Papyrus, discovered by G.M. Ebers in 1872 and allegedly written around 1500 BCE, contains a list of medical prescriptions with animal, vegetable and mineral ingredients. Each prescription includes details of the symptoms of the disease being treated and provides information on preparing and administering the cure. It is basically a herbal giving recipes and formulae for naturally derived medicines. The papyrus also contained invocations to the gods Ra, Isis and Horus, indicating the magico-religious element so important in Egyptian medicine. The ancient Egyptian healers and physicians were also magicians who were expert at exorcism and ritual; so entwined with healing were magical practices in Egypt during the rule of the Pharaohs that the folk charms and remedies which have survived there today still include prayers to the ancient gods and goddesses. In addition to herbal remedies the Egyptian physicians used charms, votive offerings, incantations, divination and religious ceremonial. In many cases supernatural origins were offered by the priesthood to explain medical conditions with which they were not familiar – rather than admit to their patients that they did not have all the answers the ancient Egyptian physician, like doctors throughout the ages, looked around for a scapegoat.

But Egyptian medicine should not be dismissed as mere superstition supported by a knowledge of medicinal plants. Physicians also carried out surgery, including circumcision. In the event of the death of the patient while being treated by a legitimate doctor, the latter could face the death penalty if found guilty of negligence. This sounds harsh, but the physician was protected: if after four days of the established medical procedure being carried out the patient showed no improvement, the physician was allowed to use alternative treatments. If, after all this, the patient still did not recover, the physician was absolved of all blame if the illness proved fatal.

Although there are numerous references to diseases in the Old Testament there seems little evidence of an organized class of physicians, folk healers or herbalists among the Hebrew tribes. In the New Testament, too, various diseases are mentioned, and one of the disciples who followed Jesus as he travelled the countryside preaching was Luke the physician. It can be surmised that by the time that Jesus began to preach his message to his fellow Jews, who were under Roman occupation, Greek culture, including the arts of the physician, had become widely diffused throughout Judea. Certainly Jesus can be regarded as a folk healer, in the widest possible sense, because he used his healing powers to help the country people. His healing ministry included exorcism to drive out evil spirits, and in that respect he had much in common with many other wandering holy men who preached radical forms of Judaism at the same time.

At the time of Jesus Greek medicine was highly developed. In ancient Greek mythology Aesculapius, or Asklepios, was traditionally the founder of medical practices. He was the god of healing who was taught the wisdom of herbs by the leader of the mythical centaurs, Chiron; in memory of this legend the term 'Chironic medicine' is sometimes given to herbalism and folk healing. In Greek mythology Aesculapius was the son born to the sun god, Apollo, and a mortal woman named Koronis. Apollo himself was said to be a god of healing, because of his solar attributes. His daughter Hygiea carried on the medical tradition, lending her name to the modern practice which is so essential in preventing the spread of infectious diseases. In common with his ancient Egyptian counterpart Imhotep, Aesculapius is said to have been originally a mortal, taught the medical arts from physicians in the Nile valley. He allegedly invented the surgical probe for the exploration of wounds, and introduced bandages and ligatures.

The Greek medical profession was organized into a separate caste or social class. They were paid an annual salary by the state, based on a municipal tax in what resembles a Greek national health service. Each physician was chosen by a public assembly, before which he had to appear and prove that he had the required practical skills to become a member of the profession. All physicians had an office in which they interviewed patients, prepared medicines and carried out operations. They employed medical assistants, who were themselves training to become doctors, and slaves who were only allowed to treat their own class. Religion still played an important role in Greek medicine, and it is recorded that before surgical operations the physician made invocations to the god Apollo.

Herbalism also featured in Greek medicine. The earliest Greek herbal was the *Codex Anicare Julianae*, which is preserved in the National Library of the Vatican. It is a sixth-century edition of a herbal written in the first century by the Greek herbalist Dioscorides. During the fourth century schools of medical science were founded, which attracted botanists and physicians from all over the Middle East. During this period of intense medical activity many new herbals were written and circulated among the healing profession.

Hippocrates, who gave his name to the ethical oath sworn by modern doctors, was one of the first Greek medical practitioners to have an impact on the healing arts. His writings included advice on diet and personal hygiene, and listed over four hundred herbal remedies for a variety of diseases. About a hundred years later another Greek physician, Theophratus, born 370 BCE, wrote his seminal work *The Enquiry into Plants*. This, the first attempt at a scientific method of botany describing common plants, was to prove very useful to medical herbalists who wanted to identify plants in their natural habitat.

It seems probable that the Romans were taught their herbal lore either from the Greeks, or from the Celts whom they conquered as they swept westwards across Europe. Pliny the Elder (*c.* 23–79 CE) was the most important writer on medical plants in ancient Roman times and devoted seven of the thirty-seven volumes of his *Historia Naturalis* to herbal lore. Unfortunately, despite its academic title Pliny's work contained fantastic details of plants and their attributes which were based only on popular superstition and folklore. For this reason it is of little use as a practical herbal, although this fact did not prevent medieval herbalists quoting from it frequently to support the medical claims for their products. Another herbal, written in 200 CE by the Greek Galen, was more accurate. He had travelled extensively and his books became the standard medical texts for Roman healers. Through their military campaigns in western Europe the Romans spread the use of Mediterranean herbs to this part of their empire. Roman officials planted herbs in their gardens which they brought from home, and many of these imported species began to grow in the wild. Fennel, dill, rosemary, savory, garlic, parsley, mustard, mint, thyme, hyssop and sage were all introduced into western and northern Europe during their occupation by the armies of imperial Rome.

Many of the sophisticated techniques employed by pagan medical practitioners were lost at the beginning of the Christian period, especially when the ancient libraries, repositories of pagan wisdom, were burnt to the ground. The collapse of the Roman Empire as a result of internal social disorder and uprisings among its conquered enemies, and the foundation of the Christian Church as the political force which replaced it, ushered in the historical period which we call the Dark Ages. During this time the scientific knowledge of the classical world, along with its major religious and philosophical teachings was rejected by the followers of the new faith.

But despite the Church's opposition to pagan medical practices there are many examples of ancient medicine being used in Teutonic and Anglo-Saxon society. The Roman historian Tacitus recorded in his book *Germania* that after a battle wounded German warriors sought out their wives and mothers, who sucked and licked the wounds. It is well known that human saliva has healing properties. In pagan Germany a special class of priestesses, known as the *Weise Frauen* or wise women, were credited with healing powers. In Scandinavia the established priesthood, known as *godi*, were often assisted by shamans, or *lahki*, who were skilled in the use of medical herbs and possessed supernatural powers to heal the sick. Shepherds, herdsmen and blacksmiths were also generally employed as healers, bonesetters and herbalists; they practised in remote rural areas where no *godi* or *lahki* was available.

Despite their conversion to Christianity, the Anglo-Saxons retained many of their pagan beliefs regarding the causes of disease. For their healing lore, the Saxon doctors drew on many sources of inspiration, including classical Greek medicine, Teutonic magic, Celtic beliefs, Roman herbalism and Byzantine occult philosophies. The combination of these different strands of knowledge comprised the Saxon art of leechcraft which was practised during the Dark Ages.

The folk healer or witch doctor in Saxon times was expected to be capable of treating a complex range of diseases and complaints. Established leech doctors were in fact practitioners of common folk medicine. They held a privileged position in Anglo-Saxon society, but were not easily identifiable because they had no particular distinguishing physical appearance or type of dress. High educational standards were not regarded as very important. Medical textbooks used by the folk doctors had been translated from Latin and Greek into Old English, so, providing they could read, the leech doctors had access to a considerable amount of information on herbs and folk remedies.

Although many of these herbals or leech books were based on early Greek, Roman and Arab treatises there is every indication that the Saxon doctors used indigenous healing practices which owed very little to external influences. The medical expertise gained by the leech doctors was passed on to their apprentices and eventually written down in the reference books consulted by literate folk healers. Evidence of any organized guild or professional body of folk medicine practitioners in Anglo-Saxon society is slim; nor does there seem to have been an established code of practice or ethical system, so obviously that was not one of the positive aspects borrowed from Greek medicine.

The collection of herbs and healing plants was accompanied by the chanting of prayers and magical incantations. Herbs were also gathered in strict accordance with the phases of the moon, a practice which survived into the Middle Ages and far later, when folk healers used occult wisdom in conjunction with herbal remedies. In medieval times the gathering of herbs at the correct astrological aspect was an important stage in folk magic rituals to heal the sick. Another Anglo-Saxon custom which has survived even today is the use of a natural measuring system which uses such phrases as 'a handful of elder flowers' or 'a pinch of caraway seeds' instead of the more scientific units of measurement. The practice of herbalism and folk remedies has always been regarded as an intuitive art – the healer works with nature to treat the mind, body and spirit of the patient.

One of the most famous folk magic charms used by Saxon leech doctors for healing combines occult lore with pagan mythology and herbalism and is known as *The Lay of the Nine Healing Herbs*:

> These nine attack
> against nine venoms
> a worm came creeping
> he tore asunder
> then took Woden
> nine magical twigs
> then smote the serpent
> that he in nine [pieces] dispersed
> Now these nine herbs have power
> against nine outcasts [unclean things]
> against nine venoms [poisons]
> against nine flying things
> [and have might] against the

loathed things
that over land rove
Against the red venom
Against the white venom
Against the blue venom
Against the yellow venom
Against the green venom
Against the dusky venom
Against the brown venom
Against the purple venom
Against the worm blast
Against the water blast
Against the thorn blast
Against the thistle blast
Against the ice blast
Against the venom blast
If only venom came flying from
the east or only from the south
over mankind
I alone know a running river
and the nine serpents behold [it]
All weels must now to herbs give
way
seas dissolve
all sea water
when I this venom
from thee blow.

This incantation contains a specific reference to the Germanic/Nordic Woden or Odin, the shamanic god who hung on the Cosmic World Tree for nine days and nine nights. As a result of this ordeal he received by divine inspiration the wisdom of the magical alphabet known as the Runes. The Saxons believed that Woden had the power to destroy the evil serpent which they believed was the originator of disease. Woden also features on a tenth-century manuscript written in Old High German which was found in Merseburg cathedral, Saxony, in Germany. Although written during a period when Christianity was the official religion, it contains open references to pagan gods indicating that the old ways still survived. The manuscript includes the following magical charm for a sprained ankle:

Baldur and Woden
fared to a wood
there was Baldur's foal's foot
sprained
Then charmed Woden
as well he knew
for bone sprain
for blood sprain
for limb sprain
bone to bone
blood to blood
limb to limb
as though they were glued.

In Norse mythology Baldur was the beautiful young god of
the sun who was killed through the trickery of Loki. In the
transitional period between Christianity and paganism Baldur
was often identified with Jesus, and this is confirmed by the
following (Christianized) version of the magic charm quoted
above.

Our Lord rade [rode]
his foal's foot slade
down he lighted
his foal's foot righted
bone to bone
sinew to sinew
blood to blood
flesh to flesh
heal in the name
of the Father, Son
and Holy Ghost.

As mentioned earlier, the Anglo-Saxons relied heavily on
herbal-based remedies in their medical cures. In addition to
their native herbals the leech doctors also had access to
translations of classical works, which included the *Herbarium
Apuleii Platonici*, an original Latin herbal dating from the fifth
century BC. The Saxon translation of this herbal, now preserved
in the British Museum, dates from 1000 BC and belonged to the
school of Aelfric at Canterbury in Kent.

The most famous native herbal of the period is *The Leech
Book of Bald*, allegedly written by a physician named Bald who

was closely associated with the court of King Alfred. In the herbal Bald refers to correspondence he has seen between Alfred and the King of Jerusalem on the subject of herbalism. The King sent Alfred a list of Syrian healing plants with their medical properties and prescriptions for their use. The herbal, of 109 leaves, was written in a large bold hand with one or two initial letters displayed in illuminated script. From its contents it can be concluded that Bald was a qualified physician with considerable medical knowledge; he refers to two other doctors, Dun and Oxa, who provided him with folk remedies that they used in their daily consultations. In medieval herbals of the fourteenth and fifteenth centuries the numbers of medically potent plants listed range from 150 to 350, whereas Anglo-Saxon herbals such as Bald's listed over five hundred.

The Saxons thought that many diseases were the work of fairies, elves and hobgoblins, a pagan belief which survived into medieval times when mental illness, for instance, was blamed on demonic possession. In *The Leech Book* the causes of many diseases are credited to the malicious actions of elves, who fired at human beings poisoned arrows – elf shot – which infected them. The concept of elves as understood by the Saxon and Germanic peoples was totally different from the gossamer-winged sprites of nursery fairy tales. The Saxon elves dwelt in the dark solitude of the forest wilderness and resented any intrusion by mankind. They were divided into two separate categories, the shining bright elves and the dark black elves. It was the latter who were held responsible for misfortune and illness; they could be kept under control only by the use of magic spells, charms and herbal remedies as presented in the Saxon medical texts used by the leech doctors.

One typical herbal recipe from *The Leech Book* is a salve to be used to ward off the elven race and nocturnal visions which cause nightmares. It was also allegedly used to help heal women who had been forced to perform sexual acts with the Devil! The recipe given by Bald is as follows:

> Take the ewe hop plant, wormwood, Bishop wort, lupin, ashthroat, henbane, harewort, viper's bugloss, heatherberry plants, cropleek, garlic, grains of hedgerife, githrife and fennel. These herbs are to be put into a vessel and placed beneath the altar where nine masses are sung over them. They are then

boiled in butter and in mutton fat, holy salt is added, the salve is strained through a cloth and what remains of the worts [herbs] is thrown into running water. The patient's feet, head and eyes are to be smeared with the ointment and he is to be censed with incense and signed over with the sign of the cross.

Today we recognize that nightmares, insomnia and disturbed sleep patterns are the symptoms of psychological disruptions in the human psyche. Within the context of Saxon leech lore the idea that they were caused by externalized spirit forces is just as valid.

Closely allied to elf shot was something called 'flying venom'. The various types of venom are listed in *The Lay of the Nine Herbs*, and were regarded by the Saxons as the agency through which diseases were passed from one person to another. According to Saxon medical opinion these venoms were carried by the wind and could be blown away by a magician or priest using incantations or a mixture of herbs, holy water and salt. This composition was sprinkled over the patient and the sickbed. Today we recognize in this ancient description of flying venom the phenomenon of disease-carrying bacteria.

One herbal folk remedy for the cure of the effects of flying venom reads:

Take a handful of hammerwort and a handful of camomile and a handful of waybroad [plantain] and roots of water dock. Seek which will float and add one eggshell full of honey, then take clean butter. Let him who will help to work up the salve melt it thrice. Let one sing a Mass over the worts [herbs] before they are put together and the salve is wrought up.

Closely interwoven elements of pagan belief and practice existed alongside the influence of Eastern and Christian religious ideas in Anglo-Saxon leech craft. They included the idea mentioned above, that some types of diseases such as mental illness, sexual perversion and epilepsy, were the result of the possession of the patient by demons or evil spirits. In such instances both exorcism by Christian priests and herbal remedies by leech doctors were employed in a joint effort to drive the occupying spirits from the body of the sick person.

In *The Leech Book* periwinkle and mandrake are singled out as plants with special powers to relieve demonic possession. In folk medicine mandrake has always been regarded as a plant with strange powers. According to medieval legends the mandrake screams when it is torn from the ground, and anyone who heard the noise was immediately struck dead. Because of this odd belief medieval herbalists employed specially trained dogs to uproot the mandrake so that they themselves escaped this terrible fate. While this folk tale sounds ludicrous, there may be an element of truth in it which has been sadly obscured by medieval superstition. Mandrakes do possess very long roots, and have been known to make a squeaking noise when they are pulled up. When periwinkle was used to cure possession by evil spirits it had to be gathered using a precise magical formula. It was picked 'when the moon is nine nights old and eleven nights old and thirteen nights and thirty nights and one night old'. Only plants collected in this way would be potent enough to exorcise demons successfully.

The Saxons grew some of the herbs they used in specially prepared herb gardens which they called *wyrtzerd*, but the majority were gathered from the wild. Herbal medicines were prepared by crushing the plants, using a pestle and mortar, and then adding them to ale, milk or vinegar. Potions were manufactured by mixing herbs with honey, and ointments were made by working herbs with butter. Herbal baths for curative purposes were also popular at this period – it was not until later that the medieval Church condemned bathing as a sin. Cosmetic recipes based on herbs were also included in the work books of the leech doctors. For sunburn it was recommended to 'boil in butter tender ivy twigs and smear therewith'. Another cosmetic preparation says 'that the body should be clean and glad and bright hue take oil and dregs of old wine equally, put them into a mortar and mingle well together and smear the body with this in the sun'.

Our Saxon ancestors also used herbs as a protection against the alleged powers of darkness, against being bitten by dogs and for safety from robbers. Herbs could be bound to different parts of the body – such as the forehead to cure head pains – by red threads, cords or wool. In Germanic mythology the colour red was sacred to the thunder god Thor, who was associated with healing and protection against evil. Red was also used in popular folklore to represent sexual energy, vitality and the life force.

In common with later medieval folk belief, the Saxons thought that disease could be transferred from the patient to inanimate objects by the use of simple magical acts. Using this process, for instance, diseases could be deflected into running water (which carried it away), or blood from an infected wound could be thrown across a wagon way or footpath. If a person was bitten by an insect or a rabid animal and the bite became infected, the practitioner of leech craft collected a few drops of blood from the wound. This was placed in a spoon made from green hazel wood. The leech doctor then went to the nearest wagon way and in complete silence threw the blood from the spoon across the path. It was believed that shortly afterwards the infection would vanish and the wound would begin to heal.

In the magic charm which was used when gathering peri- winkle the number nine was prominent. It also features in *The Lay of the Nine Herbs* as a significant number with magical properties. Its use in Saxon and Teutonic folk remedies is connected with the fact that nine is a lunar number, represent- ing the three phases of the moon multiplied by itself. In ancient magical rites of pre-Christian origin the moon was strongly featured as a symbol of the pagan Mother Goddess. The worship of this deity was a central act in the pagan Old Religion, which survived into the Middle Ages in a degenerate form under the guise of witchcraft.

The magical and pagan elements which formed such an important aspect of Saxon leech craft were regarded as quite natural by the ordinary country folk, but were not regarded with a similar degree of tolerance by the Church and its officials. Egbert, Archbishop of York, preached a sermon against the use of herbs for magical rituals, and even prohibited the harvesting of herbs if accompanied by the recitation of magical or pagan incantations – although he did add the provision that it was permitted if the end result was for 'Christian purposes', whatever they may have been. As early as 640 St Eligius had preached against herbalism in a general condemnation of the persistent survival of paganism in Saxon England.

Ye shall observe none of the impious customs of the pagans neither sorceries, nor diviners, nor soothsayers or enchanters nor must you presume for any cause to enquire of them . . . let none regulate the beginning of any piece of work by the day or the moon. Let none trust in or presume to invoke the names of demons neither Neptune or Orcus, nor Diana nor Minerva nor Geniscus nor any other such follies. Let no Christian place lights at the temples or the stones or at fountains or at trees or at places where three ways meet. Let none to presume to hang amulets on the necks of man or beast. *Let no one* make *lustrations nor enchant herbs* nor to make flocks pass through a willow tree or an aperture in the earth. For by doing so is to consecrate them to the Devil. Let none on the kalends of January join in the wickedness and ridiculous things, the dressing up like old women or like stags or make feasts lasting all night or keep up the practice of gifts or intemperate drinking. Let no one on the festival of St John [24 June] or any of the other festivals join in the dances or leaping or diabolical songs.

One of the many pagan incantations which upset the early Christians who converted the Saxons from their heathen ways was the following prayer to Mother Earth. In common with other pagan peoples the Saxons regarded the Earth as feminine and represented it in their mythology as a goddess. This prayer was commonly used in Anglo-Saxon times by the leech doctor and folk healer as they gathered herbs or prepared remedies.

Hear I beseech thee and be favourable to my prayer. Whatsoever herb thy power dost produce give I pray with goodwill to all nations to save them and grant me this my medicine. Come to me with thy powers and howsoever I may use them may I have good success and to whomsoever I may give them. Whatever thou does grant it may prosper to thee all things return. Those that rightly receive these herbs from me do make them whole. Goddess I beseech thee I pray thee as a supplicant that by thy majesty thou grant this to me. Now I make intercession to you all ye Powers and herbs and to your majesty ye who are Earth, parent of all produced and given as a medicine of health to all nations and hath put majesty upon you be I pray ye the greatest help to the human race. This I pray and beseech from you and be present here with your virtues for She who hath created you [the herb] hath herself promised that I may gather you into the goodwill of him whom the art of medicine was bestowed and grant for health's sake good medicine by grace of thy powers. I pray grant me through your virtues that whatsoever is wrought by me through you may in all its powers have a good and speedy effect and good success and that I may always be permitted with the favour of your majesty to gather you into my hands and to glean your fruits. So shall I give thanks to you in the home of that majesty which ordained your birth.

A similar magical incantation to a pagan goddess, which was evidently used by folk medicine practitioners dates from the twelfth century. A modern translation from Old English reads:

Holy Goddess Earth, parent of Nature, who dost generate all things and regenerate the world which thou alone sharest to the folk on earth. Thou guardian of heavens and sea and the arbiter of all the Gods by whose influence Nature is wrapt in silence and slumber thou art she who restoreth day and putteth the darkness to flight, who governest the shades of night in all security restraining at thy will the mighty Chaos, winds, rains and storms or letting them loose. Thou churnest the deep to foam and putteth the Sun to flight and arouseth the tempests. Or again at thy pleasure thou sendest forth the glad daylight. Thou givest us food in safety by a perpetual covenant and when our soul passeth away it is in thy bosom that we find our haven of rest. Thou too art called by the loving kindness of the Gods, the Great Mother who has conquered the God of mighty name. Thou art the force of nations and Mother of the Gods without whom nothing can be born or come to maturity. Mighty art thou Queen of the Gods! Thee O' goddess I adore in thy Godhead and on thy name do I call, vouchsafe now to fulfil my prayer and I will give thee thanks O' goddess with the faith that thou hast deserved. Hear I beseech thee and favour my prayers. Vouchsafe to me O' goddess that for which I now pray to thee grant freely to all nations upon Earth all herbs that thy majesty bringeth to life now suffer me thus to gather thy medicines. Come to me with thy healing powers. Grant a favourable issue to whatsoever I shall make from these herbs and may those thine to whom I shall administer the same. Prosper thou all thy gifts to us for to thee all things return. Let men take these herbs rightly at my hand. I beseech thee now O' goddess may thy gifts make them whole. I beseech thee that thy majesty may vouchsafe this boon.

The Church's reaction to this incantation can easily be imagined. The words explicitly invoke a pagan deity of feminine origin who is addressed as the creator and controller of the natural world, usurping the role of the Christian God as represented by the medieval clerical establishment. The use of this blatantly pagan prayer addressed to a supreme feminine principle as late as the twelfth century offers ample proof that the old ways were still actively followed and supported by ordinary people.

The knowledge of herbalism was strictly controlled by the Church during the European Dark Ages, but outside its repressive influence there was a considerable trade in its raw materials and in information on their use. Arab doctors, who had studied the great works of the Greek and Muslem physicians, made great advances in the study and practice of medicine during this period. A Persian doctor named Avicenna (980–1037 CE) wrote a treatise called *Canon Medicine* which became a standard medical textbook for Arab physicians. He had studied the properties of medicinal plants and learnt how to distil the essential oils from flowers and herbs.

At Salerno in Italy an advanced medical school was established which taught techniques based on the writings of the Greek medical profession. During the Crusades many wounded soldiers were evacuated from the Holy Land for medical treatment at this hospital. Nobles from all over Europe travelled to Salerno to pay large sums of money to receive the benefits of its medical facilities.

It was through Arab influence that Greek medicine and medical philosophy permeated European culture. In the twelfth century a group of translators became established in Toledo in Spain. They translated Arab medical books founded on Greek ideals into Latin, the universal language of medieval European academics. From Italy other sources of medical knowledge were becoming available through the writings of Constantine the African (1020–87), an Arabic-speaking Christian monk responsible for translating several important Arab medical books into Latin.

During the latter part of the Dark Ages and the early years of the medieval period the Church was gradually increasing in political power and began to persecute unofficial folk healers and herbalists. As mentioned earlier, even in its infancy the Church had felt strong enough to launch verbal attacks on the survival of paganism among the peasant population. In 314 the Synod of Ancyra had forbidden the practice of healing using occult powers. This prohibition was reinforced at the Synod of Laodicaea in 375 and reinforced by other Synods in the fifth, sixth and seventh centuries. The Church condemned all forms of healing the sick as the work of the Devil, and from the fourth to the twelfth centuries reigning popes issued decrees which prevented priests and nuns from studying medicine or administering to the sick except for the performance of the Last Rites. Despite this restriction, many clergy defied their papal leadership. In 1215 Pope Innocent III promulgated a decree which threatened to excommunicate any priest who dared to practise surgery.

This harsh attitude to medical practices gradually softened as the Church became more confident in its campaign to eradicate the surviving remnants of pagan belief in medieval Europe. In an amazing change of opinion the Church began to adopt the role of physician to its flock, using a bizarre mixture of approved magical practices and Christian theology. Pagan charms and prayers for the sick were Christianized, as we have seen, so that they could be used by priests, nuns and monks. The priesthood began to perform the laying on of hands and used exorcism rituals to drive out diseases. Patients were anointed with holy water and sacramental oil, and the cult of holy relics became popular. These were pieces of dirty rags or bones which were allegedly the mortal remains of saints and disciples. Kept locked inside clerical shrines, these relics were only exhibited in public for healing purposes or on special saints' days. Large sums of money were charged for the benefit of touching these objects. Considering the nature of these relics, many of which were blatantly faked, it seems likely that more disease was spread by their use than was ever cured. During the Middle Ages the use of relics to heal the sick became a money-making enterprise and led to many scandals within ecclesiastical circles.

Some positive results of the Church's new interest in healing were seen in the Middle Ages. The use of herbs was adopted on a large scale. Many monastery gardens boasted well-stocked herb plots, and rare plants were imported from the Mediterranean and Middle East to supplement the native varieties. The Benedictine monastic order in particular became renowned for its learning in the field of herbalism and folk medicine; its monks studied both Greek and Roman medical books in an attempt to augment the basic knowledge about medical matters which was then available. Medieval monasteries had attached to them infirmaries for the treatment of local sick people. These were the direct predecessors of modern hospitals such as St Thomas's in London. Each of these monastic infirmaries had an adjacent herb garden which would have contained such well-known plants as mustard, fennel, thyme, sage, rue, mint, parsley and pennyroyal.

Despite the fact that the Church had accepted medical practices it still regarded unorthodox practitioners operating outside its fold with a suspicion bordering on hostility. In the fourteenth century the papal authorities issued edicts against unauthorized healers including midwives, apothecaries and herbalists. In an attempt to curb the influence of rural healers in 1421 the Church prohibited women from practising medicine; if they refused to obey they were sent to prison. Pope Sixtus IV later condemned the practice of medicine by 'Jews and men and women who are not university graduates'. Even the most innocent attempt to help the sick was fraught with potential danger: in 1322 a woman was brought to court in Paris, charged with pretending to cure people of internal complaints, with treating abscesses and open wounds, and with 'examining the urine in the manner of a physician, feeling the pulse and touching the body and limbs'. Several prominent people appeared in her defence to testify that she had cured them of long-standing illnesses and one witness said that the woman had more medical knowledge than all the physicians in Paris.

When the Church began its horrific persecution of alleged witches in the late fifteenth century the position of the folk healer, herbalist and midwife became even more difficult. Anyone outside the Church who used charms or folk remedies to cure sickness became a target for the witch hunters. If found guilty, they faced long imprisonment or even death. The new laws condemning witchcraft had a dramatic effect on the practice of folk medicine: it was driven underground, and during the persecutions a considerable amount of herbal lore was lost.

In the *Mallues Maleficarum*, a guide prepared by two Dominican monks in 1486 for use by the judiciary who persecuted witches, a clear distinction was drawn between wicked and good charms – magical formulae which were the work of the Devil, and those which the Church accepted as legitimate expressions of the Christian faith, the belief in the Holy Trinity and the intercession of the saints. The book in fact recommended only the use of the Pater Noster (or Lord's Prayer) and the Ave Maria as safe charms to heal the sick. When witch hunting became a commercial business in the sixteenth and seventeenth centuries the demonologists who searched out suspects recommended burning herbs to ward off the evil spells of their quarry. Medieval theologians believed in a class of demons known as succubi and incubi, entities which appeared in human form and had sexual relations with their willing or unwilling victims. Church exorcists burnt herbal-based incense in bedrooms at night to prevent the amorous advances of these demons. This incense included such ingredients as sweet flag, ginger root, pepper, clove, cinnamon, mace, nutmeg, benzoin, resin, aloewood and sandalwood. According to one recipe, these raw materials were brewed in three and a half quarts of brandy and water. It is interesting to note that several of the herbs listed have alleged aphrodisiacal properties – a strange choice to ward off sexually aroused demons!

It was widely believed in the Middle Ages that witches had magical powers which enabled them to fly through the air. In some of the early witch trials alleged witches had claimed that they had flown to the Sabbat (the gatherings attended by covens of witches on the dates of old pagan festivals) with the aid of flying ointments made from herbal ingredients. When the Irish noblewoman Lady Alice Kyteler was accused of practising witchcraft in 1324 it was claimed that she possessed a staff 'on which she ambled and galloped through thick and thin when and what manner she listed after having greased it with ointment which was found in her possession'. Another account dates from 1435, when a woman charged as a witch said she rubbed herself with ointment and immediately fell asleep. She then had a dream in which she was flying to the Sabbat to cavort in front of the Devil with other members of her sisterhood.

Such stories led some authorities both within and outside the Church to dismiss the stories of witches flying on broomsticks as delusion. They believed that the narcotic materials in the herbs used for the witches' flying ointment entered the bloodstream of the anointed person, creating hallucinations. In the sixteenth century demonologists had sensationally claimed that the primary ingredient of the flying ointment was the fat of boiled children who had not been baptized. Such a ridiculous claim suggests a desperate attempt by the Church to encourage parents to baptize their offspring into the new faith at an early age, or face the horrific consequences of having them murdered by witches.

Francis Bacon quotes one recipe for flying ointment which contains 'the fat of children dug out of graves'; however he also lists several herbal raw materials, such as wolfbane and cinquefoil, which sound as if they might have been a genuine part of the recipe. Bacon voiced the opinion that the brew 'drugged the witches into delusions of flight'. This experience was, he claimed, caused not by incantations but by anointing themselves with the herbal ointment. Another person with scientific knowledge, Henry More, stated in 1653 that the use of the flying ointment by 'filling the pores keeps out the cold and keeps in the heat' which sounds a sensible conclusion. One active ingredient in the flying ointment was either bear or goose grease, which suggests that the witches used it to keep warm while performing naked outdoor rites.

Several folk recipes for witches' flying ointment have survived. Among the herbs used in their composition are aconite, which changes the rate of the heartbeat, and belladonna (deadly nightshade), which caused delirium. There are three typical recipes: parsley, water of aconite, poplar leaves and soot; water parsnip, sweet flag, cinquefoil, bat's blood, deadly nightshade and oil; baby's fat, juice of water parsnip, aconite, cinquefoil, deadly nightshade and soot. Bat's blood was obviously included because of that animal's ability to fly at high speeds and to sense in the dark. Soot was added presumably because it would make the witch less visible at night.

In 1545 André Lagina, the personal physician to Pope Julius III, was involved in the arrest of a couple accused of witchcraft in the French province of Lorraine. He discovered hidden in the couple's house a jar filled with green liquid, examination of which showed it to be composed of narcotic herbs such as hemlock, deadly nightshade, henbane and mandrake. Lagina tested the liquid on the wife of the local city hangman; on being anointed with the herbal brew, she fell into a deep sleep with her eyes open 'like a boiled hare'. The Pope's physician tried to wake her without any success, and she remained in a comatose condition for thirty-six hours. When she finally regained consciousness she was angry at the physician, for she told him he had taken her away from 'all the pleasures of the world'. Turning to her husband, she said, 'Knavish one, know that I have made you a cuckold, and with a lover younger and better than you.'

Modern authorities on witchcraft have attempted to test the authenticity of these medieval accounts of the flying ointment. In 1902 Karl Kieswetter, a German scholar fascinated by the occult, made a sample of the ointment using a traditional recipe. After rubbing it into his skin he fell asleep and dreamed he was flying through the air in a spiral motion. Another researcher, Gustav Schenk, experimented with henbane by burning the seeds and inhaling the resulting smoke. He reported feeling dizzy, had the feeling that his body was becoming lighter and that parts of his body, including his feet and head, were growing larger. As the intensity of the experience increased Schenk thought that his body was falling apart and felt the sensation of flying at high speed through the air.

One of the most interesting accounts of the witches' ointment was reported by Dr Erich Peuckert, a professor at Göttingen University, in 1960. Dr Peuckert had been studying psychic phenomena and the occult for over forty years and was fascinated by the folk tales of witches flying on broomsticks. In a book called *Magia Naturalis*, or *Natural Magic*, written by Johannes Baptisa Porta in 1568, he discovered a formula for the flying ointment which included thornapple, henbane and deadly nightshade. The original recipe called for baby fat, but the professor substituted ordinary lard from his local grocer. Dr Peuckert decided to experiment on himself and chose a close friend whom he could trust to be his assistant. At six o'clock one evening the two men retired to a private room in the university where they knew they would not be disturbed. They applied the ointment to their wrists and forehead, as suggested in the book. Within a few minutes they had fallen into a deep, trance-like sleep which lasted over twenty hours. When the doctor and his assistant awoke they had the symptoms of a severe alcoholic hangover including violent headaches, sore throats and dry mouths.

Independently, each wrote down a detailed account of his experiences while under the effect of the ointment, and then compared notes. Both men reported sensations of flying through the air, and both had visions of demonic faces. Dr Peuckert reported landing on a hilltop where he indulged in erotic rites with naked women and paid homage to a creature who looked like traditional representations of the Devil.

As a result of his experiment with the flying ointment, Dr Peuckert firmly believed that medieval witches really thought they had flown to the Sabbat and indulged in weird rites. The hallucinogenic nature of the herbs used in the salve, and the ignorance of the peasants, would have prevented them from distinguishing fact from fantasy. The majority of confessions obtained from alleged witches were based on evidence given under torture, which would have increased the sense of unreality.

According to the professor, the secret knowledge of hallucinogenic herbs may have been introduced into medieval Europe by the wandering bands of gypsies who originated in India. This knowledge was disseminated by groups of wise women, who had knowledge of herbs which could both cure and kill, and whose secret societies were the remnants of the matriarchal priestesshoods of the pagan Old Religion. Peuckert also believed that those who used the ointment reported similar experiences because the natural chemicals in the herbs stimulated areas of the brain responsible for creating access to atavistic racial memories of pagan rites.

The witch trials naturally concentrated on the more sensational aspects of the craft. Although the rural herbalists, folk healers and charmers were the targets, along with survivals of pagan customs and practices, at the height of the anti-witchcraft hysteria thousands of innocent people were murdered by the legal authorities. In 1592 a Catholic priest called Father Loos said, 'Wretched creatures are compelled by the severity of torture to confess things they have never done. By cruel butchery innocent lives are taken and by a new alchemy gold and silver are coined from human blood.'

By the early seventeenth century the charge of witchcraft was not only being made against the poorest and uneducated members of society but had extended to include the higher social levels. A canon of Trier cathedral in Germany reported that those burnt at the stake for the alleged practice of witchcraft included a judge, two burgomasters, several councillors and a parish priest. The executioner made so much money out of his bloody work that he rode around like a noble at court on a white horse and clad in gold and silver.

Despite the ferocity of the witch hunt the profession of herbalist and folk healer survived in rural areas of the English countryside. The persecution in England generally did not reach the same peak of hysteria as it had done on the Continent. Even so, during the period 1558 to 1736, when witchcraft ceased to be a major crime, it is estimated that at least 1800 people were executed as alleged witches. The peak period for the witch hunt in England seems to have been, predictably, during the puritanical times of the Commonwealth after the Civil War and, perhaps more surprisingly, during the reign of Queen Elizabeth I.

Each village had its wise man or woman who was skilled in the use of herbs and other forms of folk healing. Often the female wise women were also midwives and laid out the dead. In their role as local midwife they knew which herbs could be safely used as painkillers during childbirth. Ergot, a fungus derived from yeast, was used as a pain reliever at a time when clerics taught that the pain of childbirth was God's punishment on women for the original sin commited by Eve in the Garden of Eden. Wise women also used fresh dung to treat open wounds. Initially our modern reaction to this drastic treatment might be one of horror and disgust, until we consider that both dung and spider's webs, also used to cover wounds, are natural sources of penicillin. They also used willow bark to cure headaches, several hundred years before doctors discovered that it contains the natural source for the ingredients of the modern aspirin. While physicians were still prescribing blood letting and magical charms for curing the sick, the rural wise women had developed an extensive knowledge of herbal remedies and natural drugs which they used to alleviate the misery of many otherwise incurable diseases.

Evidence that the herbal remedies of the country folk healers were not just superstitious mumbo-jumbo is offered by the true story of Dr William Withering (1741–99), who discovered the cardiac stimulant known as digoxin. The doctor found out that the local people in rural Shropshire often preferred to consult wise women who offered folk remedies rather than visit his surgery. One old lady was universally renowned for a herbal tonic she brewed, which had proved successful on many occasions for treating heart conditions. Dr Withering visited the witch and, after lengthy negotiations, purchased the recipe for her miracle cure. When he analyzed the remedy he found that it contained foxgloves or digitalis – the origin of the modern drug digoxin. In his book *An Account of the Foxglove* Withering stated that he had identified twenty different herbs in the potion, but foxglove was the most potent of them all.

The wise women and folk healers also recommended the chewing of raspberry leaves or the drinking of raspberry tea for period pains and childbirth. Modern scientific tests have proved that the leaves of the raspberry plant contain a natural substance which relaxes the uterus. The white witches, as these benign witches were called, also used nettles as a blood purifier. Today it has been discovered that the nettle plant contains a large concentration of vitamin K, which helps to prevent excessive bleeding.

Village wise women were frequently the only people to whom the sick could turn in time of need. In 1552 Bishop Latimer stated: 'When we are in trouble or sickness or lose anything we run hither and thither to witches and sorcerers whom we call wise men seeking aid and comfort at their hands.' Such learned men as Elias Ashmole, founder of the Ashmolean Library at Oxford, and the famous diarist Samuel Pepys believed in the efficaciousness of magical spells to cure illness. Ashmole wore three dried spiders to ward off attacks of the ague, and Pepys always carried a hare's foot around his neck to prevent colic. Most of the popular healing charms used in the sixteenth and seventeenth centuries to cure various diseases were based on Christian prayers, mixed with Hebrew incantations borrowed from the Jewish mystical tradition known as the Cabbala and the grimoires, or grammars, of medieval magic. Other magical charms from this period can be directly traced back to the Anglo-Saxon leech books.

As mentioned earlier, it was still a widely accepted belief among some rural folk healers that many illnesses were caused by the malicious influence of ghosts, black witches and fairies. In some cases the so-called cunningmen were also witchfinders, who would seek out some harmless old woman and accuse her of bewitching their patients. Such anti-social reactions were a direct result of the Church's propaganda relating to the activities of witches in rural communities, accusing them of bewitching livestock and ruining crops with their spells.

Other folk healers actually practised witchcraft as defined in the narrow sense by the Church and the legal officers responsible for justice in country areas. Joan Warden was accused of practising the craft in 1592 merely because she 'not only used charms but doth use ointments and herbes to cure divers diseases'. A Yorkshire woman called Alice Morton was brought to trial for practising witchcraft because she admitted curing cattle with remedies; she denied, however, that she ever cast spells on them to make the animals recover. A woman arraigned before a court in Aldeburgh, Suffolk, in 1597 was said to 'take upon herself to cure diseases by prayer and therefore have recourse of people to far and wide'.

During the sixteenth, seventeenth and eighteenth centuries the wise woman had an important role to play in village society. As well as the folk healers who specialized in herbal remedies, every housewife was expected to have some knowledge of natural treatments for common ailments. An old book dated from the early eighteenth century, when witch hysteria had abated, states that the housekeeper should have 'a competent knowledge of physick that they be able to help their maimed, sick and indigent neighbours for commonly all good and charitable ladies make this a part of their housekeeper's business'.

This social responsibility to act as a healer to the local community was not restricted to servants. Wealthy and aristocratic women were widely expected to learn the use of folk remedies to help those less fortunate than themselves. According to one eighteenth-century writer, a wealthy woman should help her neighbours who are too poor to purchase the assistance of a physician. Those who did not have access to a gentlewoman with healing skills relied on the services of the traditional practitioner of folk medicine. One writer referred to these wise women in the following terms: 'I do not mean to speak of the old woman at [Stoke] Newington beyond St George's Fields unto all the people resort as an oracle, neither will I speak of the woman on the Bankside who is as cunning as the house of cross keys nor yet of the cunning woman in Seacole Lane who have more skill on her cole basket than judgement in urine and knowledge in physic and surgery'.

In the medieval period the practice of medicine, by both orthodox physicians and the village wise men and women, was inextricably linked with magical practices and occultism. Towards the close of the Middle Ages one of the leading proponents of the magico-occult approach to treating disease was Phillipus von Hohenheim (1493–1541), popularly known as Paracelsus. He was not only widely versed in occult lore but was also one of the most enlightened medical exponents of his age. Born at Enseiden in Switzerland, he was the son of an eminent medical student who had become a practising doctor at Villach in Austria. When Paracelsus was a young boy his father often took him on expeditions to the Alps to locate rare herbs which were used for medicinal purposes. The impact of these field trips caused the boy to study medicine as a young man, and in 1515 he received his doctorate in medical science at the famous school for physicians at Ferrara in Italy.

Paracelsus had always been interested in the hidden side of life, and this now led him to study the occult; he pursued his lust for knowledge in that area by adopting a nomadic lifestyle and wandering around Spain, Italy, Greece, Sicily and Russia. In each place he discovered further information about medical practices, with which he complemented the techniques he had learnt at Ferrara. He also studied at many of the leading European universities, published books and exchanged ideas with the most learned men of his time. As well as developing contacts with the highest levels of the academic world Paracelsus delved into the underworld of witches, gypsies, folk healers and herbalists. From these people he discovered the secrets of herbal cures, folk charms, magical rites and such occult arts as palmistry and the tarot.

Paracelsus became convinced that diseases originated in the three substances which the alchemists believed formed the material universe, and which were symbolized on the physical level as salt, sulphur and mercury; in occult terms they represented the mind, body and spirit. If these three aspects of a person are in perfect harmony with each other, then Paracelsus believed that no disharmony or dis-ease could exist. If the three aspects are not balanced, which is frequently the case, then disease manifested itself in the physical body as a direct result of this imbalance. This concept may have seemed far-fetched in the sixteenth century, but today it forms the basis of holistic medicine, including herbalism, which is gradually becoming more acceptable. Even orthodox members of the medical profession have now recognized the link between mental attitudes and common illnesses such as cancer, asthma, heart disease, influenza and stress.

Within the three kingdoms or realms represented by salt, sulphur and mercury Paracelsus identified five causes of disease. He categorized these as, firstly, those from the *Ens Astrale* or created by causes in external nature (environmental factors); secondly, those from the *Ens Veneri* or poisons and impurities (pollution); thirdly, those from the *Ens Naturae* or causes derived from the parents (hereditary diseases and genetic disorders); fourthly, *Ens Spirituale* or those caused by morbid imaginings or evil will (psychological states); and, lastly, *Ens Dei* or those created by the will of God, which could be a legacy from previous existences experienced by the human soul and manifested in this life as a form of divine justice (karmic disease).

One of the most interesting aspects of Paracelsus's definition of disease and its origins is the category known as *Ens Veneri*. He believed that if anything entered the constitution of a human being which was not in harmony with his or her elements 'the one is to another an impurity and can become a poison'. While orthodox medicine tends to deal only with external affects and physical causes, the type of esoteric or occult medicine practised by Paracelsus and many folk healers searched for the fundamental effects which were the cause of the physical symptoms.

As an example of this process at work, according to the theories of Paracelsus promiscuous sexual activity not only increased the risk of sexually transmitted diseases but could also have psychological complications. A person who indulged in physical relations with a sexually deviant man or woman could, according to Paracelsus, be affected with both mental and spiritual malaise. He believed that during the act of sexual intercourse the spirit essence of the partners blended. Any form of sexual act with another person creates a transference of emotional, mental and spiritual energy, which, depending upon the circumstances, can have either a beneficial or a malefic effect on the partners in the act. Sex can therefore be a mystical healing experience or exactly the opposite. It is the difference between established partners making love and the sexual violence between a rapist and his victim.

Paracelsus also believed that changes in the phases of the moon, the influence of the planets and their movements and differences in climatic conditions and atmospheric pressure could have an affect on human wellbeing. He supported the occult doctrine that mankind is a microcosm within a macrocosm – a tiny replica of the universe. Physical changes in material conditions could therefore have an adverse effect on human health. If he were alive today, Paracelsus would have no difficulty in accepting the modern idea that negative and positive ions in the atmosphere can effect human behaviour; he would also have accepted the recent theory put forward by scientists that comets could be responsible for the outbreak of virus infections on Earth. Paracelsus also taught that thought transference was taking place all the time between people who lived or worked in close proximity. Because of this he claimed that some diseases, especially those of a psychological or psychosomatic nature, could be transmitted from one person to another purely on a mental level.

Controversy naturally surrounded Paracelsus wherever he went. His claim that astrology could be used as a diagnostic tool in medicine was ridiculed by the new breed of physicians who wanted to divorce medical matters from what they regarded as medieval superstition. Paracelsus's friends, the witches, gypsies and folk healers, had taught him the assignation of the zodiac signs to the anatomy of the human body; they had also instructed him in the manner by which various diseases could afflict a person if certain planets were badly aspected in their natal horoscope. To diagnose illness Paracelsus utilized, too, the occult arts of physiognomy (the study of character defects by the features of the face or the form of the body) and cheiromancy (examination of the lines in the palm of the hand). These aspects of occult wisdom were denounced in the sixteenth century as sorcery, but he insisted that by studying lines of illness in the face or discoloured patches of skin he could identify the nature of the illness affecting his patient and prescribe the required course of treatment.

Paracelsus was a pioneer in the field of sixteenth century medicine who sadly was not recognized by his medical contemporaries. He realized that the mentally ill were not sinners possessed by demons but very sick people in desperate need of specialized treatment. He studied the links between disease and the environment of the patient, which had received medical prominence only in recent times. He noted, for instance, that miners often suffered from bronchial problems, and traced this directly back to daily contact with coal dust. He also advocated sunlight, fresh air and frequent baths to speed recovery from long illnesses – this was at a time when sick people were locked away in darkened rooms on the orders of orthodox physicians.

This radical doctor laid down stringent rules which dictated the criteria by which a genuine medical practitioner should be judged – rules designed to cleanse the profession of the many charlatans and quacks who preyed on the gullible, extorting large sums of money from the wealthy for their cranky treatments which were often highly dangerous. In the wise words of Paracelsus, 'A good physician should possess a clear conscience, a gentle heart and cheerful spirit. He should lead a moral life and have a greater regard for honour than for riches. In all matters he should seek to be more useful to the patient than himself.'

Against a background of general ignorance in medical matters in the sixteenth century Paracelsus stands out as a liberal influence seeking to revolutionize the treatment of disease and the relationship between the doctor and his patients. Naturally enough, these enlightened views were not widely accepted, and Paracelsus was criticized by both the orthodox medical community and the fraternity of charlatans who saw in his radical proposals a threat to their income. In desperation at the frequent and savage attacks on his character he once remarked bitterly, 'This pack of mad dogs which attacks me is so large but its understanding is so small.' At one stage the persecution became so concentrated that Paracelsus was forced to walk the streets as a beggar in order to escape physical attack. He clothed himself in rags, slept in ditches and survived on scraps of food donated by charitable passers-by.

While Paracelsus was a compulsive traveller who seldom stayed in one place for more than a few years before moving on, he did manage to find time to write several very important books. His most famous medical works consist of eleven treatises on well-known diseases such as tuberculosis, colic and worms; despite the general opposition to his occult theories, these books became standard reading for sixteenth-century physicians. In addition to medical books he also penned philosophical works including *De Generatione Hominis* or *The Origins of Man*, which dealt with his personal theory of cosmology, and *De Vita Longa*, on hermetic alchemy.

Despite his study of the occult Paracelsus was conventionally a very religious person and remained a practising Catholic throughout his life. He did, however, draw philosophical inspiration from the semi-pagan Gnostics of the early Church, the ancient Greeks and the medieval Jewish Cabbalists. He told his pupils that if they wished to study the inner life of humanity they must learn to examine the foundation of nature as expressed through the teachings of the Cabbalistic mystics. He argued that the Cabbala embraced the ancient occult sciences of astrology, alchemy and mysticism, which the discerning student could use to unravel the spiritual side of reality through their symbolic interpretations. Anticipating Jungian psychology, Paracelsus taught that any disturbance experienced by the inner self created psychic ripples which were the root cause of physical illness.

Because of his investigation into the psychic realms and the occult, Paracelsus was the subject of persecution by the Church despite the fact that he was a dedicated Catholic. He was accused of signing a pact with the Devil in exchange for forbidden knowledge; in the sixteenth and seventeenth centuries this was a common form of slander used against original thinkers who advocated anti-Establishment or anti-clerical ideas which did not meet with the approval of the Pope.

It was hoped that by labelling a person as a devil worshipper he would be made a social outcast by his peers and be unable to propagate his radical ideas. The Church capitalized on the fact that Paracelsus had studied alchemy, the art of transforming lead into gold – which was an occult metaphor for the transformation of matter into spirit – by claiming that he had bargained the so-called elixir of life from the Devil. This elixir had allegedly granted the Swiss physician the gift of immortality, a nonsensical claim disproved when Paracelsus died at Salzburg in 1541. Even after his death the legend of the magical powers which Paracelsus was supposed to have possessed during his lifetime persisted. When bubonic plague swept through Salzburg it was reported that hundreds of people knelt at the doctor's tomb, praying for a cure.

Paracelsus was not alone in seeking advice or inspiration from the rural herbalists and folk healers. Orthodox physicians who had been using herbs for centuries had learnt their craft from the village wise men and women and put it into practice in the cities. During the medieval period the first herbals published since the Anglo-Saxon leech books began to appear in limited editions. The first major work in English on botanical medicine was the *Rosa Medicinae* or *Rosa Anglica*, written in the fourteenth century by a monk called John of Gaddesden. It was based on Greek, Arabic, Jewish and Saxon sources, but also included original data collected by the author.

The invention of printing in the late fifteenth century provided access to a considerable amount of new information on herbalism which boosted its study despite the disapproval of the Church. By the beginning of the sixteenth century many original works were being produced, with printed illustrations of all the plants listed. The first authentic printed herbal is believed to have been written by John Banckes in 1525. In 1550 an English physician named Anthony Askham published an enlarged edition of the Banckes herbal and attributed the actions of herbs to astrological correspondences. The most influential of these early printed herbals was *The New Herball*, written by William Turner and published in 1551; it was based on Turner's travels around Europe studying botany, and the cultivation of herbs in his garden at Kew. John Gerard's three-volume *Herball*, published in 1597, became one of the standard reference works of the period. Born in 1542, Gerard was head gardener to the influential Cecil family during the reign of Elizabeth I. He was also a member of the Company of Barber Surgeons in the City of London; in those days barbers were also surgeons and bloodletters – they gave enemas, performed amputations and extracted teeth. The traditional red and white striped pole which used to be a feature outside old-fashioned barber's shops was a reminder of their original duties.

Gerard's herbal is still in print today, and another reference book on herbalism which has survived the passing of time is the one written by Nicholas Culpeper (1616–54). The son of a clergyman, while still very young Culpeper acquired a considerable knowledge of Latin and Greek. At the age of eighteen he went to Cambridge, and while at the university fell in love with a young heiress. Culpeper persuaded her to elope with him, and they planned to get married in the Sussex town of Lewes. They travelled to their secret destination separately, but the young woman's coach was struck by lightning during a fierce thunderstorm and she was killed instantly. This tragic event completely shattered Culpeper's life. He abandoned his studies at Cambridge and became an apprentice apothecary in St Helens, Bishopsgate in the City of London. After a very short time the brilliant student, still only twenty-four, began his own practice as a medical herbalist in Red Lion Street, Spitalfields. The same year he married Alice Field, a girl of fifteen with a large fortune. His career in Spitalfields was disrupted by the Civil War, during which he fought on the Royalist side and was wounded in the chest by a musket ball. This injury was to lead to tuberculosis, which eventually caused his early death.

As an apothecary and medical herbalist Culpeper was very unorthodox in comparison to other physicians of the period. His strong belief in astrology drew ridicule from his medical contemporaries, who thought that Culpeper was following the example of the rural folk healers. Although he expressed an interest in occult matters, Culpeper made a considerable contribution to the advancement of medical expertise. During his comparatively short career as a physician he had privately printed many tracts on medicine. Although condemned by his critics, they sold well to the general public and helped to dispel some of the ignorance about medical matters which existed in the popular mind. In contrast to the bigoted attitude of his contemporaries, the public recognized in Culpeper a person who was not afraid to be outspoken and who was willing to court unpopularity from his peers for the benefit of the common people.

In 1649 Culpeper translated *The Pharmacopoeia*, the standard reference book in Latin for apothecaries issued by the College of Physicians, and published it, with his critical comments, as *A Physicall Directory*. Culpeper's motive in providing this translation was his personal conviction that medical information should be freely available and not restricted to the upper-class élite. The reaction from his colleagues in the medical profession was swift and predictably virulent: they resented any attempt to remove the aura of mystery which obscured medicine from the masses. The publisher, on the other hand, was very pleased with the venture, for it became a minor bestseller. Culpeper was encouraged to write more books, and the one which gained him the most success was *The English Physician*, published in 1652, two years before his death.

He will always be remembered, however, not for the scholarly textbooks he wrote on conventional medicine but for his famed *Herball*, which in 1986 is still in print in a popular edition. Subtitled 'A compleat physick whereby a man may preserve his body in health and cure himself being sick for three pence charge with such things as grow in England, they being most fit for English bodies', it lists over four hundred different common plants with medicinal uses giving their description, healing actions, astrological correspondences and recipes for their use to cure illness. It is truly a phenomenal work which, although heavily criticized for its superstitious content, has proved invaluable to generations of herbalists and their patients. Orthodox physicians who were incensed by the publication of the *Herball* denounced it as having been produced 'very filthily by two years drunken labour corrupting men's minds with his opinions beside the danger of poisoning men's bodies'. The fact that it is still being consulted today by many herbalists and folk healers offers proof that this statement is untrue.

Originally, apothecaries like Nicholas Culpeper were merely peddlers of drugs which they purchased from others. Gradually, however, the apothecaries became skilled in the preparation and use of natural drugs. The term 'apothecary' comes from a Greek word meaning 'storehouse', and in Roman times an *apotheca* was a place where medicinal herbs were stored. The title of apothecary was given to the keepers of these stores. Many royal palaces and noble households in the Middle Ages had a resident herbalist, who was first known as the spicer or pepperer but later adopted the title of apothecary; his job was to administer the herbs, spices and perfumes used in the household. In fact the office of court apothecary had an unbroken history from early medieval times – the court records of 1313 mention one Odin the Spicer, who was in the pay of King Edward II. He was paid 7½*d* a day to be apothecary to the Queen. Early apothecaries obviously had other royal duties, for in 1329 one was paid to embalm the body of Robert the Bruce. The earliest English reference to an apothecary is in 1180, when one accompanied King Henry II to Ireland. Another apothecary was mayor of York in 1213, and in the same city in 1292 an apothecary was established called Otto the German.

In the fifteenth century the apothecaries became associated with the Grocers' Company in the City of London, which was a medieval guild. The guilds had been set up as early trade unions to protect the legal rights of various types of tradespeople, craftsmen and artisans. Apothecaries were also usually members of the College of Physicians, which had been founded in 1518 by royal charter. The College insisted that no medical practitioner within London and seven miles around could practise unless he had been examined and approved by the Bishop of London or the Dean of St Paul's.

The apothecaries usually purchased their herbal raw materials from the so-called 'Green Men' or 'Green Women', rural folk healers who wandered the countryside collecting herbs for use in remedies. Eventually many apothecaries established their own herb gardens in the towns and cities to grow supplies of medicinal plants. Orthodox physicians disapproved of the contact between apothecaries and the exponents of traditional folk medicine, and in 1540 an Act was passed giving the College of Physicians the legal right to enter an apothecary's shop, examine his wares and, if they considered them unsafe, have them destroyed. By the late sixteenth century the apothecaries had ended their association with the Grocer's Company and formulated plans to establish a separate guild in the City of London which would be responsible for their interests. In 1617 the Worshipful Society of Apothecaries of London was founded, with an initial membership of 114. At the same time an Act of Parliament was passed forbidding grocers and surgeons to prepare or sell medicines. Among established medical practitioners the apothecaries therefore now possessed a monopoly for supplying herbal remedies and medical drugs.

These seventeenth-century apothecaries were the lineal descendants of the old herbalists of the Middle Ages and, through their contact with the rural-based healers, preserved many of the tenets and practices of folk medicine. Their reason for leaving the Grocers' Company was the widespread malpractice which permeated orthodox medical treatments at this time. In the opinion of the new apothecaries' guild,

> unskillful and ignorant men do abide in the City of London which are not well instructed in the art or mystery of Apothecaries but do make and compound many unwholesome, harmful and deceitful, corrupt and dangerous medicines and the same do sell and daily transmit to the great peril and daily hazard of the lives of our subjects. We therefore weighing with ourselves how to prevent the endeavours of such wicked persons thought necessary to disunite and disassociate the apothecaries of the City of London from the freemen of the Mystery of Grocers into one body corporate and politic to whom in all future times the management of these inconveniences might be given in charge and commited after the manner of other companies.

This breakaway movement by the apothecaries was deeply resented by the Grocers, who rejected the charges of misconduct made against them and sought to restrict the new company. However, James I interceded on behalf of the apothecaries and granted their society a royal charter which effectively established them in the City as a respected guild with equal rights to all the others. In response to the granting of the King's charter the apothecaries insisted on strict membership qualifications to deter charlatanism; they even seized dangerous drugs or fraudulent medical products which they saw offered for sale and had them destroyed. It was recorded that one persistent offender was fined the sum of £6 13s 4d for selling 'bad drugs' called 'Methridatic' and 'London Treacle'. Such products were usually burnt in public before the door of the offender.

One of the leading members of the Society of Apothecaries was Thomas Johnson, who was responsible for producing an enlarged edition of Gerard's *Herball* and presented the Society with a copy for its library. Johnson is also said to have been the first person to bring bananas to London. To the amazement of passers-by, he displayed a bunch of these tropical fruits in his shop window on 10 April 1633. Johnson had obtained them from his friend Dr Argent, President of the College of Physicians, who had brought them back from a trip to the West Indies. It was Johnson who introduced the Society to the idea of field trips into the countryside around London to the then rural hamlets of Piccadilly and Islington, to Hampstead Heath and Kent, to gather wild flowers and herbs with healing powers.

From the late 1600s to about 1750 the role of the apothecary as a professional medical practitioner gradually increased. The day book of an unnamed apothecary in Shrewsbury, dated 1706, relates that he sold over the counter to casual customers an assortment of gargles, mixtures, ointments and patent medicines made from herbal ingredients. He also supplied essential oils, gums, spices, resins, chemicals such as saltpetre and borax, soap, brushes, varnish, ink and pencils. In addition to herbal remedies some apothecaries sold coffee, tea, candied oranges and lemons, jam and biscuits, reflecting their earlier membership of the Company of Grocers.

The medical ingredients offered in the *London Pharmacopoeia*, which were available to physicians at this time, make an interesting comparison with the naturally based products sold by the apothecaries. The *Pharmacopoeia* listed nearly two thousand remedies in common use, whose ingredients included dried worms, fox lungs, oil of ants, live frogs, moss from the skull of a murder victim, crabs' claws, saliva from a fasting man, human placenta, snakeskin, swallows' nests, woodlice and the powdered bones of an executed criminal.

In 1673 the Society of Apothecaries had rented from Lord Cheyne four acres of land by the Thames at Chelsea. A full-time gardener was employed in the new garden and plants were transferred from the already well-established Westminster Herb Garden. The garden in Chelsea was walled, and Lebanon cedars were planted for the first time in Britain at the gate nearest the river. During the next two hundred years the Chelsea Physic Garden, as it came to be known, became famous as the repository of herbs from the English countryside and more exotic plants from overseas. The garden created by the seventeenth-century apothecaries is still in existence, and every year is visited by over three thousand botanists and herbalists from all over the world.

During the three hundred years when the apothecaries were establishing their role as the forerunners of nineteenth and twentieth-century doctors the country folk still relied on the skills of the village wise men and women when they fell ill. Their use of traditional folk remedies brought them into conflict with those who held orthodox views. Midwives, who were often also folk healers who used herbal preparations, were especially singled out. In the sixteenth century the Church had persuaded Parliament to rule that all midwives had to be licensed by their local bishop before they could practise. It also prohibited the use of magical charms, prayers and incantations. Midwives had traditionally also christened babies, but the Church ruled that they should only use plain water as opposed to consecrated water and not indulge in 'profane words'. In the late seventeenth century several midwives were accused of witchcraft because, in contradiction of clerical regulations, they used charms to ease difficult births.

Traditional folk medicine had already been dealt a hard blow in 1512 by an Act which condemned 'ignorant persons of whom the great part have no manner of insight or any kind of learning . .·. common artificers as smiths, weavers and women boldly and continually take upon themselves great cures and things of great difficulty in which they partly use witchcraft and sorcery'. Although officially the use of herbal and folk remedies was outlawed, we know from the profusion of apothecaries and their support by the highest in the land that such authorized types of folk medicine were accepted. Henry VIII, for instance, was very interested in folk remedies and had his court physicians prepare over two hundred ointments, medicines and balms which were based on the herbal recipes of folk healers. Charles II and a number of other monarchs also practised an unorthodox form of healing known as 'the King's touch': he would lay his hands on a sick person and say 'I toucheth thee but God dost healeth thee'. A gold coin was then hung around the person's neck by the king, and he or she was presented with 7s 6d. This royal healing ritual was performed within the sight of a priest, who blessed the proceedings.

The hypocrisy of the double standards in judging medical expertise was obviously noted by Henry VIII's counsellors, for in 1542 the original Act of 1512 was amended to exclude from prosecution a category of folk healers described as 'divers honest persons whom God hath endowed with the knowledge and the nature, kind and operation of certain roots, herbs and waters and the using and ministering of them to such as He provided with disease'. Presumably this amendment was made to prevent apothecaries from facing court appearances for selling remedies based on herbs. It also gave greater freedom to the rural wise men and women who, in theory, could practise their healing craft without fear of prosecution by the law and interference from the Church.

Any euphoria the wise men and women might have felt at this turn of events was quickly dissipated by the passing of the 1563 Witchcraft Act, which reinforced the law prohibiting the use of charms and incantations to heal the sick. Even with this severe restriction in operation the wise men and women still managed to ply their trade, and were consulted by both rich and poor alike – occasionally they only escaped prison because of patronage by wealthy clients. One sixteenth-century wise woman was saved from prosecution because she had treated Sir Francis Walsingham, the head of the 'secret service' and confidant of Elizabeth I.

As the number of trained doctors increased, so the role of the village wise woman began to alter as a result. The first sign of this change was the loss of many of their wealthy patients who abandoned folk remedies for the new methods offered by the apothecaries and physicians. During the eighteenth and early nineteenth centuries the rural wise women and folk healers were increasingly consulted only by poorer members of the community who could not afford to pay for medical attention. Those people who were on a low wage and unable to buy medicines had otherwise to rely on the voluntary support offered by those hospitals that had been set up as charities. This inequality led to a resurgence of interest in herbalism and folk remedies during the nineteenth century. Numerous self-help medical books were published which offered recipes and information for curing a wide variety of common ailments; many of these remedies were based on traditional folk medicine. As late as 1910 an official government report stated that the wise women were still active in country districts where they sold salves, ointments and charms for the treatment of abscesses, sores and burns. It was not until the inauguration of the National Health Service in 1946 that their role began to decline in the face of free medical attention for all and improved facilities for dealing with the sick. However, as can be seen by the recipes collected in this book, traditional folk medicine still played an important part in the lives of many country people until comparatively recently.

Some of the folk remedies practised in the eighteenth and nineteenth centuries seemed to have been based on the worst aspects of medieval superstition. For curing rheumatism country people wore the skin of an eel as a garter, for headaches they wore a snakeskin, and they believed that sore eyes could be cured by washing them with rainwater that fell on 1 June. In the *Sussex County Magazine* of 1939 Dr P.H. Luham reported that even as late as the 1930s local people took their babies to wise women to cure them of diptheria, which was done by tying a hazel twig around the infant's throat; the cost of this treatment was 1s, and if it failed the unfortunate baby had to swallow a piece of stewed mouse, for the price of 2s 6d. *The Brighton Herald* of 1835 records the case of a woman cured of a wen on her hand by the touch of a corpse. For tuberculosis, snails or slugs were boiled up in a broth in milk and eaten before breakfast. An eighteenth-century recipe for 'Snail Water', used in treating various ailments, ran:

> Take a peck of garden snails, shells and all. Wash them in spring water. Bruise them in a stone mortar. Steep in 3 gallons of best ale. Add hartshorn, raspberry, 6 ounces of bruised clover, 2

ounces of liquorice, half a pound of aniseed, 1 ounce of cinnamon, 1 ounce of nutmegs. Let it steep day and night. Distill on a slow fire.

Other strange beliefs in the nineteenth century included wearing a large spider around the neck to cure ague, a superstition which seems to date from the 1600s. For fevers and nosebleeds, country folk wore a toad around their throats. To cure eyestrain, folklore recommended a poultice of crushed snails and bread. In the nineteenth century Sussex folk healers prescribed a live spider boiled in butter to cure jaundice. In Yorkshire a trout laid on the stomach of a sick child was said to cure colic and worms. To avoid cramp, the afflicted person was told to wear an eelskin wrapped around the left leg above the knee. A piece of wood from a gibbet or the paw of a mole carried in a velvet or leather pouch was said to be a sure remedy for toothache. In Shetland a person suffering from ringworm rubbed the affected part of the body with ashes each morning until the condition eased. While rubbing on the ashes the following rhyme was recited:

> Ringworm, ringworm, red
> Never may thou spread or speed
> But aye grow less and less
> And die away among the ashes.

As in Anglo-Saxon times, it was generally believed by country folk that illnesses could be disposed of by transference, the most common example of which is the curing of warts. In one cure, a piece of meat was rubbed on the unsightly wart and then buried in the ground. As the meat rotted away beneath the earth, so it was believed that the wart would gradually fade away.

A snail rubbed on a wart and pierced was also said to make the growth vanish as the creature rotted. In Westmorland old country people counted the number of warts, put into a small bag the same number of pebbles and dropped the bag at a crossroads. Whoever ventured by and was unlucky enough to pick up the bag inherited the warts, which were transferred through the pebbles. An alternative method of wart charming was to tie as many knots in a length of hair as there were warts and then throw it away. Or you could cut an apple in half, rub the warts with it and then tie it together again. The united apple was then buried, and as it rotted away so the warts would disappear.

In another folk remedy people suffering from ague unwound onto a tree a piece of rope which they had coiled around their body. They then ran round the tree singing,

> Ague, ague, I thee defy.
> Ague, ague to this tree I thee tie.

In cases of whooping cough the child was told to handle three live snails; they were then hung up in the chimney, and when they died it was believed the cough would go. Alternatively a spider was held over the head of the child and the following words were recited:

> Spider as you waste away
> So the whooping cough no longer stays.

The spider was then sealed in a bag and hung up over the hearth until it expired. A caterpillar, placed in a bag which was then hung round the child's neck, was used in the same way. In Sunderland the crown of the child's hair was cut and hung on a bush or small tree; birds would carry off the hair to line their nests, taking the cough with them. For a swollen throat a live snake was placed in an airtight jar. As it died and decayed the swelling in the throat would decrease.

Some folk remedies were based on the magical law of correspondences and sympathetic magic. The belief that a mole's paw hung round the neck cured toothache may have arisen because moles have sharp teeth which are good at gnawing. Similarly, babies who were teething could be helped by hanging a rabbit's paw or a dried shrew around their neck. Following the same idea powdered human skulls were used to cure epilepsy, which is a disease of the brain, and marrow or oil extracted from human bones was recommended for treating rheumatism, a disease of the bones. The slimy substance exuded by snails was dropped into the ear as a cure for earache and catarrh, presumably because it resembled nasal mucus; this was also the reason why country folk anointed the chests of children suffering with bronchitis with butter. Children in Dorset were passed through the cleft of an oak tree to cure ruptures, and those suffering from rickets were passed between two straight trees growing close to each other.

Medieval prayers also survived as charms to drive away illness. This one is for healing an inflamed wound caused by a thorn.

> Our Saviour Jesus Christ was of pure virgin born
> And he was crowned with a thorn.
> I hope it may not rage or swell,
> I trust in God it may do well.

It was believed that diseases could be cured merely by reciting words which had special religious significance, or simply by the laying on of hands. These charms and blessings were often passed down through families, preserved on pieces of paper kept in the old family Bible. One example from the Welsh border, recorded in the 1930s, is said to have been an instant cure for toothache:

> Jesus came to Peter as he stood at the gates of Jerusalem and said unto him, 'What does thou here?' and Peter answered, 'Lord my teeth do ache,' and Jesus answered him saying, 'Whosoever do carry these words in memory with them or near them shall never have toothache any more.'

Another folk charm, from nineteenth-century Herefordshire, was said to have the power of curing ague:

> When Jesus saw the cross where he was to be crucified he began to tremble and shake. The Jews asked him, 'Are you afraid or do you have the ague?' Jesus answered them and said, 'I am not afraid, neither do I have the ague. Whoever wears this [the cross] about them shall not be afraid nor have the ague.'

One of the most famous of these Christian folk charms is the following, which is found all over the country as a cure for burns.

> There were three angels came from the west
> One brought fire and the other brought frost
> The third brought the book of Jesus the Christ
> In frost, out fire
> In the Name of the Father, Son and Holy Ghost
> Amen.

Other non-religious folk charms included the curing of bronchitis by wearing a necklace of blue beads. A sore throat, too, could be relieved by wearing a blue stocking around the neck. It is interesting that blue is regarded by spiritual healers as the colour for healing and the life energy. In the 1840s, on the other hand, a shop in London's Fleet Street sold what were called 'Red Tongues' – small pieces of red cloth which were purchased by people as a cure for scarlet fever, presumably because of their colour.

Although today we may laugh at the more bizarre examples of folk remedies, some of the cures were found to have a use in orthodox medicine. One famous example is cod liver oil, officially introduced in 1772 by a Manchester doctor as a treatment for rheumatic pain; it had been widely used by sailors and fishermen for the same purpose for several centuries.

Even as late as the nineteenth century the plant lore used as the basis for herbal remedies was still influenced by the so-called Doctrine of Signatures, devised by Paracelsus in the sixteenth century. According to this Doctrine, if a plant resembled a particular disease or complaint then it was believed to have the power to cure it. If a particular plant resembled a part of the human anatomy in shape, colour or habit, then it was popularly said to be able to heal any disease which affected the organ it resembled. Writing about the general theory of the Doctrine of Signatures, the famous herbalist William Turner said, 'God hath imprinted upon the plants, herbes and flowers as it were in heiroglphicks the very signatures of their virtues.' According to Kircher,

Since one and all the members of the human body under the wise arrangement of Nature agree or differ with the several objects in the world of creation by a certain sympathy or antipathy in Nature it follows there has been implanted in the providence of Nature, both in several members and in natural objects, a reciprocal instinct which impels them to seek only those things which are similar and consequently beneficial to themselves and to avoid and shun those things which are antagonistic and hurtful. Hence has emanated that more recondite part of medicine which compares the signatures or characteristics of natural things with the members of the human body and by magnetically applying like to like produces marvellous effects in the preservation of human health. In this way the occult properties of plants – first of those endowed with life and secondly of those destitute of life – are indicated by resemblances for all exhibit to men, by their signatures and characteristics, both their powers by which they can heal and the diseases in which they are useful. Not only by their parts (as the root, stem, leaf, flower, fruit and seed) but also by their actions and quantities (such as their retaining or shedding leaves, their offspring, number, beauty and deformity, form or colour) they indicate what kind of service they can render to man and what particular members of the human body to which they are specifically appropriate.

Using the Doctrine as a guideline, spotted and scaly plants were believed to be able to cure skin complaints, perforated herbs were recommended for open wounds, plants exuding juices or resins were good for sores, plants that swelled up could be used to treat tumours, and those that shed their bark or skin were ideal for cleansing the skin. Any herb or plant which resembled blood, phlegm or bile was said to be able to cure diseases which create these bodily by-products. Herbs such as lungwort, which is spotted with dark scars, were used to treat tuberculosis and other lung diseases. Liverwort, so named because it resembles the liver in its shape, was used for the treatment of all liver diseases and complaints. Bloodroot was named after the red colour of the roots, and was specifically used for treating bloody discharges and internal bleeding. Canterbury bell or throatwort was, as its common name suggests, recommended for sore throats, possibly because it has a very long stem or neck. Plants which grow between stones and in rockeries – such as saxifrage – are reputed to be able to break up kidney and gall bladder stones. Forget-me-not, whose flower spike is suggestive of a scorpion's tail, is recommended for insect bites. The silky fronds of maidenhair are recommended for curing baldness. According to William Turner,

Walnuts have the perfect signature of the head. The outer husk or green covering represents the pericranium or outward skin of the skull whereon the hair groweth. Therefore salt made of these husks or barks are exceedingly good for wounds of the head. The inner woody shell hath the signature of the skull and the little yellow skin or peel that covereth the kernal of the hard meniga and piamater are the thin scarfes that envelope the brain. The kernal hath the very figure of the brain and therefore it is very profitable for the brain and resents the poison.

Although some herbalists today regard the Doctrine of Signatures as the outdated product of medieval superstition, it has been found that in practice plants which resemble a certain part of the body are capable of healing disorders which affect that area.

Today the herbal remedies of our ancestors have received a new type of respectability with the interest in alternative therapies and holistic medicine. These new types of medical knowledge, often based on ancient techniques, approach the subject of illness from a different angle from the one taken by orthodox medicine. They are interested in treating the whole person, taking diseases and illnesses as examples of the way in which the mind, body and spirit of the patient manifest disharmony in the total system. Herbalism, which was derived from the old folk remedies, is today a very sophisticated branch of alternative medicine which is increasingly winning scientific recognition and acceptance. In the United Kingdom alone there are an estimated four thousand medically qualified herbalists who have been legally recognized within the provisions of the 1968 Medicines Act.

The importance of the herbal ingredients in folk remedies has been investigated by several scientific research institutes, including Harvard University who amassed a vast collection of data on the subject which revealed totally new information for use by doctors, scientists and botanists. Similar work on folk remedies has been undertaken in West Germany, with the assistance of rural folk healers, in Eastern bloc countries, China, Japan, India, the Netherlands and in other universities in the USA. Research into the efficaciousness of folk remedies and their herbal ingredients has been carried out in the United Kingdom under the auspices of the Herb Society, which has founded a national herb centre with a botanical garden and has begun work on producing a computerized data bank on herbs and their medical properties.

Publication of the research data on folk remedies and herbal-based cures has revealed some interesting facts. Garlic and other plants in the onion family, for instance, have been shown to be able to reduce drastically the amount of cholesterol in the bloodstream. As we now know cholesterol is a steroid alchohol found in body cells and fluids, which has been identified as one of the causes of hardening of the arteries and may lead to fatal heart attacks. An excess of cholesterol can be created by a dependance on rich dairy product-based diets. Other discoveries made by the orthodox medical community indicate that liquorice is more beneficial for the treatment of gastric ulcers than any of the chemically based drugs currently available. Scientists have also isolated an ingredient in cayenne pepper which has proved to be a helpful natural stimulant in the treatment of nervous disorders. Recently a potential anti-cancer agent has been isolated in the common periwinkle, and, since (according to a recent article in the *Guardian*) only an estimated 5 per cent of plants have had their medical properties scientifically investigated, there are probably many more similar revelations to be found in the realm of herbal lore and folk remedy.

Our ancestors may well have shrouded herbal lore in the mist of magical ritual, but this was for a reason. Many of the plants used in folk remedies were highly toxic and their misuse would have been fatal. The legends and myths which grew up around some of the healing plants acted as a protection to prevent their abuse by the ignorant. Today, with our advanced scientific knowledge, we are beginning to realize the full extent of the medical expertise which was possessed by the folk healers, and how we can learn from their approach to healing and the techniques which they employed. In traditional folk remedies we have a legacy of ancient medical knowledge which it would be foolish to ignore or dismiss as mere rural superstition.

For all the tremendous breakthroughs made since the end of the Second World War in the field of drug therapy and medical technology, we are still faced with diseases which afflict large numbers of the human race and for which we have, as yet, no scientifically derived answer. Further research into herbal lore and folk remedies may well be the path to the answers we are searching for in orthodox medicine.

Part Two

Folk Remedies
for Common Ailments

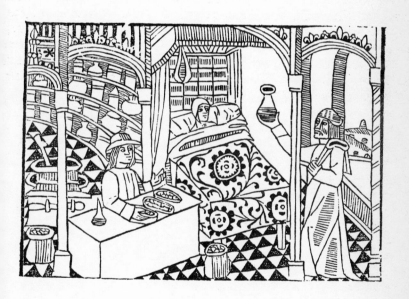

The majority of these remedies are based on herbs, the stock-in-trade of the rural medical practitioner. In contrast to the more dubious items used in folk remedies, which seem as if they belong more to *Macbeth*, the healing plants offer a comparatively safe course of medical treatment if used with care and knowledge or under the guidance of someone well versed in their usage. Before attempting to make up any of these remedies, please read for each plant ingredient the notes on application and use that are given in Part Four. They will tell you which plants should be used with caution.

The oldest remedies given here are derived from old medical literature dating back to the fifteenth century. Some were collected on the Isle of Anglesey in North Wales and date from the eighteenth century. Yet others are contemporary, and have been passed down to their present recipients as a family tradition. They are based on local knowledge, inherited wisdom and folklore, which offers proof that in the British countryside the old lore of healing plants has not been destroyed by the technological pressures of our modern age. Many of the remedies I have collected from country people all over the British Isles, and to those who participated in this two-year research project I am very grateful.

The plants are listed under the specific disease or illness which it was claimed they had the ability to heal. This enables the reader quickly to identify the appropriate remedy for his or her particular condition. Where instructions are given to add a tablespoon or teaspoon of herb this refers to it in its powdered form.

Acidity
Take 2 teaspoons of cider vinegar and mix with 1 teaspoon of lemon juice and 1 teaspoon of potato juice. Add the resulting mixture to ½ cup of warm water. Drink as required.

Acne

Take 2 oz of clover flowers, 2 oz of nettle tops and 2 oz of bonesett [comfrey] flowers. Mix the herbs together with 4 pints of boiling water. Simmer until only 2 pints are left. For the best result take 1 wineglass of the resulting liquid every 3 hours.

Ague (Malarial Fever)

Take an infusion of marigold flowers.

An ointment made with the crushed leaves of elder is also effective.

Anaemia

Dandelion tea is recommended.

Nettle tea (rich in iron) can also be taken, with 1 teaspoon of honey as a natural sweetener.

Alternatively eat raw parsley, or add ½ oz of it to 1 pint of boiling water. Strain, and take the resulting liquid 3 times a day.

Appetite, Lack of

Take a handful of hop and caraway seeds to make a refreshing drink: the seeds should be steeped in boiling water and the resulting liquid taken as required. This mixture is especially recommended after a debilitating illness.

Asthma

Agrimony tea is recommended, prepared as follows. Steep 1 oz of agrimony in 1 pint of boiling water. Strain, and take ½ cup of the resulting liquid as required.

Alternatively, garlic can be used. Macerate 1 lb of sliced garlic into a vessel containing 2 pints of boiling water. Cover, and leave for 12 hours. Add 1 oz of sugar to the strained liquid. Take 1 teaspoon at a time, as required.

Another folk remedy is to boil ¼ oz of caraway seeds and ¼ oz of fennel seeds in a vessel containing ½ pint of vinegar. When this mixture has simmered for a short time add 1½ oz of sliced garlic. Cover the vessel and leave to cool. Strain the resulting liquid and mix with 8 oz of honey. Take 1 teaspoon, as required.

An old country recipe to relieve asthma tells you to drink 1 pint of cold water every morning and to take a cold bath every two weeks.

Arthritis
Make a poultice of fresh young ragwort leaves and apply as hot as you can bear it.

A recipe for a herbal tea which is recommended for arthritic pain requires 2 oz of agrimony, 2 oz of bogbean, 2 oz of burdock, 2 oz of yarrow and ½ oz of raspberry leaves. Place the herbs in 4 pints of boiling water. Simmer slowly until only 2 pints are left. Cool and strain. Drink 1 wineglass of the liquid every 3 hours.

Another recommended folk cure is honeysuckle tea. Loosely fill a teacup with honeysuckle flowers. Add them to 1 pint of boiling water. Steep and strain. Take 1 wineglass of the liquid every 3 hours.

Alternatively take 1 handful of coltsfoot and boil it in milk with oats and butter. Apply as a poultice to the place where the pain is worst.

Backache
Make a poultice from hot aniseed and nettle leaves and apply direct to the afflicted spot.

Baldness
Rub your head with a mixture of onion juice and honey morning and evening.

Bed-wetting
It is well known that bed-wetting has a psychological or emotional cause. However for temporary relief of the unpleasant symptoms the following remedies can be tried.

Add 1 teaspoon of thyme to 3 teaspoons of honey. Take 1 hour before going to bed.

The following recipe is also recommended. Mix together ½ oz of basil, 1 oz of betony, 1 oz of golden rod and ½ oz of tansy. Place in 2 pints of boiling water. Simmer for 15–20 minutes, and cool. Take 1 wineglass every 3 hours.

A tea made from St John's wort and plantain is also suggested by folk healers. Steep 1 teaspoon of each herb in 1 cup of boiling water. Sweeten with honey as required. Take 2–3 cups a day.

Boils
Pick the centres of some blackberry shoots. Boil them, and then add cold water. Leave to soak for 5 minutes. Strain, and take 1 small wineglass of the liquid every morning.

Alternatively, heat the root of dock plant in boiling water. Strain, and drink 1 eggcup of the liquid every morning. This purifies the blood, preventing the outbreak of boils.

See also Skin Complaints.

Bronchitis
Every hour take liquorice and honey mixed in hot water with lemon juice.

According to rural folklore the following is a sure cure for bronchitis. Take 1 oz of coltsfoot, 1 oz of elderflower, 1 oz of elfwort [Elecampane] and 1 oz of white horehound. Mix the herbs into 2 pints of boiling water. Simmer down to 1 pint. When cool, add ½ teaspoon of cinnamon. Mix well. Strain, and drink 1 wineglass every 3 hours.

Another folk remedy said to produce good results is a mixture of cayenne pepper, honey and warm water. Take morning and night until the symptoms ease.

See also Coughs.

Breasts and Nipples, Soreness of
Take 1 oz each of camomile flowers and bruised marshmallow roots. Boil in 2 pints of water until it has reduced to 1 pint. Place the roots and flowers in fine linen and use as a poultice on the breasts.

Alternatively take equal parts of vervain, betony and agrimony. Pulverize and mix with beer. Strain, and add the resulting liquid to boiling milk. Drink warm to relieve breast and nipple inflammation.

Anoint the breasts with the juice extracted from a mixture of groundsel and daisies.

Take 1 oz of alum, 8 oz of sugar, 2 tablespoons of vinegar and 2 teaspoons of salt. Simmer over a low heat until a salve is created, which should be spread on a linen cloth just large enough to cover the affected breast. Leave this on until the soreness heals, then wash the breast in a mixture of warm water and milk.

If you have persistent soreness or lumps in the breast see your doctor without delay.

Breath, Shortness of

Take 1 oz of caraway seeds, 1 oz of aniseed, ½ oz of liquorice, 1 large nutmeg and 2 oz of sugar. Pulverize finely and take a pinch morning and evening.

Bruises

Make a poultice with vinegar and bran and add oatmeal or breadcrumbs. Apply to sprains and bruises for instant relief of pain and swelling.

Boil some comfrey leaves, set aside to cool, and then strain. Bathe the bruise with the resulting liquid to reduce swelling.

Take equal amounts of feverfew, ribwort, plaintain, garden sage and bugle. Pulverize them and boil in unsalted butter or vegetable oil. Strain, and apply to the bruise.

Boil a handful of hyssop leaves in a little water until tender. Wrap them in a piece of fine linen and apply to the bruise as a poultice.

Gather a handful of mallow leaves. Crush, and mix with butter or vegetable fat. Smear on bruises to stop pain and reduce swelling.

Infuse a handful of rosemary leaves in 1 pint of boiling water. Cool. Add the white of 1 egg and 1 teaspoon of brandy. Apply as a lotion to the bruise.

Burns

To produce a salve take equal parts of the root of yellow dock and dandelion, and add equal amounts of greater celandine and plantain. Extract their juices by steeping the plants in cold water. Strain carefully, and simmer the resulting liquid with a little fresh butter or vegetable fat until the butter or fat has melted. Cool, and place the liquid in containers for future use.

Peppermint oil, elderflower and marigold applied to burns can bring relief.

Take 2 pints of cream or vegetable fat and a handful of fern leaves. Boil the leaves with the cream or fat, and simmer. Allow to cool, strain, and apply to the burn.

Cancer
A tea made from steeping red clover tops in boiling water was used by country people for cancerous growths.

Catarrh
The best cure as recommended by folk healers is to eat a raw onion every morning and evening.

Alternatively, mix equal quantities of elderflowers, peppermint and yarrow. Add 1 oz of the mixed herbs to 1 pint of boiling water.

Take cinnamon and lemon juice in warm water every 3 hours.

Mix the following herbs to make an effective tea: 1 oz of coltsfoot, 1 oz of mullein, 1 oz of sage, 1 oz of thyme and ½ oz of yarrow. Place the herbs in 2 pints of boiling water. Simmer until only 1 pint remains. Take 1 wineglass every hour for the first day, then every 3 hours afterwards until the condition eases.

Chilblains
Mix 1 lb of elderflowers with 1 lb of lard or vegetable fat. Boil together and then simmer gently for 1 hour. Strain and apply the resulting liquid to the chilblains.

Bathe the chilblains in the water drained from boiling potatoes, as hot as you can stand it.

Nettle juice applied directly to chilblains eases their discomfort.

For instant results, boil an onion and apply it directly to the chilblain.

Childbirth
Six months before the birth drink raspberry tea. Add 1 oz of raspberries to 1 pint of boiling water. According to old folk belief this tea enriches the expectant mother's natural milk and prevents a miscarriage.

During pregnancy take linseed tea. Soak 1 tablespoon of linseed in 1 pint of boiling water and add honey to sweeten.

Chills
An eighteenth-century recipe for chills affecting the back and

kidney regions says slice ½ a large nutmeg into a glass of sherry or white wine. Take as required.

Colds

As would be expected, there are numerous folk remedies for treating colds. Here are some of the best ones.

Rub on the chest oil made from rosemary.

Take a handful of yarrow, ½ oz of bruised ginger root and 1 teaspoon of cayenne pepper, and add to 3 pints of water. Boil down to 1 pint. Add honey to sweeten if required. Take a glass at bedtime and repeat each evening until the cold has gone.

Take 5 lb of fresh elderberries. Simmer with 1 lb of brown sugar until it is the consistency of honey. Strain and bottle. Take 1–2 tablespoons in hot water at bedtime.

Wash your feet every evening with hot water. Then mix crushed garlic bulbs and white horehound and smear this mixture on the soles of your feet before going to bed.

Gather some fresh heads of elderflower and a handful of angelica leaves. Steep in boiling water for 10 minutes. Strain off the resulting liquid and add honey to taste.

See also Sore Throats.

Colic

Boil a handful of betony in white wine. Strain, and drink the resulting liquid for relief.

Constipation

Take honey and water every morning.

Mix slippery elm with equal parts of warm water and honey. Take morning and night.

Mix equal parts of buckthorn, rhubarb root and fennel. Boil in hot water, strain and cool. Take 1 wineglass after each meal as a laxative.

Corns

Wash the feet in hot water with some salt added. Squeeze celandine juice on to the corn and leave to dry.

Apply to the corn equal parts of apple and carrot juice plus some salt.

Apply crushed ivy leaves daily, and within a week the corn will drop off.

Coughs

As with colds, there are many folk remedies for treating coughs. Here is a selection.

Take the juice of ½ lemon, 1 teaspoon of glycerine and 1 tablespoon of honey. Fill a glass or cup with hot water, stir in the ingredients and drink as required to ease the cough.

Take 2 handfuls of coltsfoot leaves, 1 oz of garlic and 4 pints of water. Boil down to 3 pints. Strain, and add to the liquid 8 oz of brown sugar. Simmer gently for 10 minutes. Take ½ cup as required.

Take equal parts of white horehound, marshmallow leaves, hyssop, mullein and ground coriander. Infuse 1 teaspoon of mixed herbs in a cup of boiling water for 10 minutes. Sweeten with honey if required. Take 1 cup 3 times a day before meals.

Place 1 large cup of linseeds with a small quantity of liquorice and 4 oz of raisins in 2 pints of water. Simmer slowly until 1 pint remains. Add 4 oz of brown sugar, 1 tablespoon of rum and 1 tablesoon of vinegar or lemon juice. Warm ½ pint of this decoction and sip before going to bed each night.

Take 2 handfuls of coltsfoot leaves and 12 handfuls of plantain leaves. Cut and beat well. Strain the juice and add an equal amount of brown sugar. Boil to a syrup and take 1 teaspoon as required.

Thinly slice 3 garlic bulbs into a ½ pint basin. Add 4 oz of honey and ¼ pint of vinegar. Place the basin in boiling water and leave for 30 minutes. Strain off the liquid, add an equal amount of brandy, and place the resulting liquid in sealed bottles. Mix 2 teaspoons with 1 teaspoon of water and take morning and night.

Pour 2 pints of boiling water on 2 handfuls of coltsfoot leaves. Sweeten with honey. Strain, and take 3 times a day.

Take 4 oz of coltsfoot stalks and soak them in ½ pint of water. Cut the stalks into 1 inch lengths, place them in a saucepan and add some brown sugar. Stir until the sugar dissolves. Bring to the boil and skim, then reboil again until the mixture thickens. Strain the liquid through muslin into sterilized jars. Take 1 teaspoon 3 times a day.

Melt 1 teaspoon of butter or vegetable fat in a saucepan, add 1 tablespoon of honey and stir well. Add 15 drops of vinegar, stirring all the time. Take the resulting mixture 3 times a day.

Mix ½ pint of hyssop, water, ½ ounce of almond oil, 2 oz of sugar and 1 teaspoon of hartshorn. Take 1 tablespoon morning and night.

Take ½ tablespoon of dried sage and ½ tablespoon of ginger. Mix with 1 tablespoon of brown sugar. Add ½ pint of boiling water. Leave for 5–10 minutes, strain, and then sip slowly.

Add 1 tablespoon of dried sage to a saucepan containing 1 pint of boiling water. Simmer for 30 minutes. Strain, then add 1 tablespoon of vinegar and 1 tablespoon of honey. Mix well and allow to cool. Take 1 teaspoon as required.

Mix the juice of 3 leeks with the breast milk of a nursing mother. Drink 3 times daily.

Take 2 oz of caraway seeds. Boil in 2 pints of water until only 1 pint is left. Strain off half the liquid, sweeten with brown sugar and add 1 wineglass of rum or brandy. Take 1 small wineglass of the mixture every night before going to bed.

Cramp
For relief, massage into the cramped muscles clove oil diluted with olive oil.

Alternatively, crush calamint leaves, and massage the aching muscles with them.

Cystitis
Take 1 handful of dried blackberry leaves. Crush, and add them to 1 pint of water. Boil for 5 minutes, then leave to infuse for 10 minutes. Strain, and drink 3–4 cups of the resulting liquid between meals daily.

Diabetes
Mix 1 oz of agrimony, 1 oz of cloves, 1 oz of dandelion root, 1 oz of juniper berries and 1 oz of parsley, then place them in 4 pints of boiling water. Simmer until 2 pints remain. Take a wineglass of the resulting liquid every 2 hours.

Diarrhoea
To 2 pints of blackberry juice add 1 lb of brown sugar, 1 tablespoon of cloves, 1 tablespoon of mixed spice, 1 tablespoon of cinnamon and 1 tablespoon of nutmeg. Boil together for 10 minutes. Add a wineglass of whisky, rum or brandy. Bottle

while hot, cork tightly and seal. Take 1 small wineglass as an adult dose or ½ small wineglass as a child's dose 3 times a day until symptoms ease.

Mix 1 tablespoon of slippery elm and 1 tablespoon of honey with warm water and drink every hour until the condition eases.

Mix 1 oz of mint, 1 oz of queen of the meadow [Meadowsweet] and 1 oz of St John's wort into 4 pints of water, then bring to the boil and simmer until 2 pints remain. Honey, cinnamon or ginger can then be added. Drink 1 wineglass every hour.

Add 1 oz of bearberry, 1 oz of peppermint and 1 oz of raspberry leaves to 2 pints of boiling water. Simmer until 1 pint remains. Strain, and take 1 wineglass every 3 hours.

See also Dysentery.

Dizziness
For curing frequent dizzy spells drink sage tea sweetened with honey.

Alternatively, take 1 lb of fresh cowslip flowers and infuse in 1½ pints of boiling water. Add honey to taste. Simmer and take as a syrup 3 times a day.

Dysentery
Take 2 large nutmegs, 20 white peppercorns, 20 cloves, 1 oz of cinnamon and 1 oz of oak bark. Boil these ingredients in 6 pints of milk. Strain, and divide the resulting liquid into 4 equal parts. Give the patient 1 part every 6 hours for 24 hours.

Earache
Bathe the ears with a strong decoction of camomile.

For fast relief of earache, boil a large onion until it is soft and rub it on the inside of the ear.

Take a branch of young green elder and place it on a grill above a low fire. Collect 1 eggcup of the sap which will exude from the wood. Add to it 1 eggcup of fresh leek juice. Mix together well, and anoint the infected ear 3 times a day.

Eczema
Use marigold tea to alleviate the symptoms. Add 1 oz of

marigold flowers to 1 pint of boiling water. Steep, strain and take as required.

Mix 1 tablespoon of lemon juice and 1 tablespoon of honey with a pinch of cayenne pepper in warm water. Take every morning before breakfast.

Eyestrain

If you are suffering from puffy or tired eyes an old folk remedy is to apply a raw potato to the eyes, which helps to reduce the swelling.

For tired eyes, boil a handful of elderflowers in water. When cool, strain and use the liquid to bathe the eyes.

Take 1 oz of raspberry leaves, 1 oz of marshmallow leaves and 1 oz of groundsel leaves. Mix in 1½ pints of boiling water, and simmer until 1 pint remains. Allow to cool, then strain and use as an eyewash.

Blend some butter or vegetable fat, honey and the white of an egg and anoint the affected eye with it.

Anointing the eyes with the breast milk of two different women is an old folk cure for eyestrain.

Flatulence

Take a handful of feverfew, 1 oz of cumin seeds and 1 oz of ginger. Add to 6 pints of water, bring to the boil and simmer down to 3 pints. Strain and take 3–4 wineglasses a day.

Gallstones

Cut a large handful of leeks. Place them in a saucepan and cover with 4 pints of water. Cover the saucepan and simmer the water down to 2 pints. Strain off the liquid and drink a ⅓ pint of it morning, noon and night. Half the quantity can be used as a child's dose. Make up the leek water freshly every 2 days.

An eighteenth-century recipe needs 4 pints of best white wine, 2 oz of nutmegs and 2 handfuls of hawthorn flowers. Infuse them overnight in a closely covered pot. Next day, distil in a cold still, letting the liquid drop on 1 oz of sugar candy. Drink a tea dish of about 6 large spoonfuls, says the recipe, when the pain begins.

Gout

Steep some rosemary leaves in boiling water. Apply to the afflicted part of body as a poultice.

Take 1 handful of holy thistle and 1 handful of angelica leaves. Infuse, and drink ½ pint of the strained liquid every morning for a month.

Mix goose grass, tansy, sage, columbine and mint. Pound them to a fine powder, mix with beer and drink 3 times a day.

Haemorrhoids

See Piles.

Hayfever

Steep 1 oz of elfwort in 1 pint of boiling water. Strain, and take 1 small wineglass of the liquid every 4 hours until the symptoms ease.

Headache

Bathe the forehead and temples with hot water in which mint and sage has been steeped.

Take 1 small handful each of centaury and feverfew and add 1 oz of camomile flowers. Mix in 4 pints of water. Boil down and simmer to 2 pints. Add 1 oz of rhubarb while the liquid is hot, and stir well. Take 1 wineglass of the resulting liquid 3 times a day.

Take 1 oz of fresh or dried rosemary. Infuse in 1 pint of hot water. Cool and strain. For persistent headaches take 1 wineglass 4 times a day.

A fifteenth-century recipe says make a distillation of vervain, betony and wormwood and wash your head in it 3 times a week to keep away head pains.

Add ½ oz of camomile to 1 pint of boiling water. Strain, and take 1 wineglass 3 times a day.

Add 1 oz of elderflowers to 1 pint of boiling water. Strain, and take 1 wineglass twice a day.

Add 1 oz of limeflowers to 1 pint of boiling water. Strain and take 1 wineglass 3 times per day.

See also Migraine.

Heart Trouble

Add 2 teaspoons of dried hawthorn leaves to 1 pint of boiling water. Steep and strain. Add honey to sweeten if required. Take 1 wineglass 3 times a day.

Take 1 handful of centaury and boil it in beer. Strain the herbs from the beer and pulverize them. Boil again, and strain the liquid through a fine linen cloth. Mix the resulting liquid with twice the amount of honey; boil and cool. Drink 1 wineglass 3 times a day.

An eighteenth-century recipe says take as much of the herb called Dick Tender as will fill a little bag, and add it to a pennyworth of saffron dried and rubbed. Sprinkle it with salt and dry it over a chaffin dish of coals. Lay it on the heat and a warm cloth upon it. Soak the herbs in water and take the liquid 3 times daily.

Hysteria

Mix 1 oz of camomile, 1 oz of valerian, 1 oz of limeflowers and 1 oz of St John's wort and add to 1 pint of boiling water. Steep and strain. Take 1 wineglass 3 times a day.

Take 1 handful each of mugwort, red fennel and red mint. Boil in beer and strain through a fine linen cloth. Drink 1 wineglass warm 3 times a day.

Indigestion

Take 1 oz of greater yellow gentian, 1 oz of bruised columbine roots and 1 oz of camomile flowers. Add to 6 pints of water, boil and simmer down to 3 pints. Strain and cool. Take 1 wineglass 2–3 times a day.

Influenza

Mix 1 oz of boneset, 1 oz of mullein, 1 oz of sage, 1 oz of vervain and 1 oz of yarrow and put them in 4 pints of boiling water. Simmer gently until 2 pints of liquid remain. Strain and cool. Take 1 wineglass every 3 hours until the symptoms ease.

Add ½ oz of elderflowers, ½ oz of peppermint and ½ oz of yarrow to 1½ pints of boiling water. Strain, and leave for 10 minutes. Add honey to sweeten if required and drink.

Take 1 handful of angelica roots and boil gently for 3 hours in 2 pints of water. Strain off the liquid and add sufficient honey to make a syrup. Take 2 teaspoons at night before going to bed.

Insomnia
Take honey in milk with a pinch of nutmeg or cinnamon before going to bed.

Jaundice
Pulverize 1 handful of dandelion flowers, 1 handful of blue cornflowers and 1 handful of parsley in some beer. Take 1 teaspoon with food morning and evening.

Boil 1 oz of agrimony in 1 pint of water. Strain and cool. Take 1 wineglass 3 times a day.

Boil 1 oz of cinquefoil in 1 pint of water. Strain and cool. Take 1 wineglass a day.

Kidney Disorders
Boil 1 handful of nettle leaves in water. Strain through a muslin cloth. Ferment to make nettle beer. Add honey, brown sugar, cloves and ginger root. Drink 1 wineglass 3 times a day.

Mix equal parts of lime water and pearl barley water. Take 1 teaspoon 3 times a day.

Take 1 oz of burdock seeds, 1 oz of dandelion, 1 oz of marshmallow root and 1 oz of tansy. Mix the herbs well and put them in 4 pints of boiling water. Simmer until 2 pints of water remain. Strain and cool. Take 1 wineglass every 2 hours for the first day, then every 3 hours on successive days.

Lactation, Excessive
A poultice of crushed horseradish applied to each breast is an old folk remedy to prevent excessive lactation in nursing mothers.

Lung Disease
Take 1 handful of elderflowers and 1 handful of wood sorrel. Boil in milk. Strain off the liquid and take as required.
See also Tuberculosis

Migraine
Finely crush leaves of basil and feverfew. Mix well and use as snuff.
See also Headaches.

Nausea
Mix 1 handful of rosemary leaves with an equal amount of honey, and eat as required to prevent sickness.

Neuralgia
Add ½ pint of rosewater to 2–3 teaspoons of white vinegar to make lotion. Apply to the afflicted part of the body 3 times a day, using a clean cloth each time.

Nosebleeds
A nettle leaf placed on the tongue or pressed against the roof of the mouth was an old folk remedy for curing nosebleeds (presumably because the shock of the nettle sting in the tender part of the mouth stopped the flow of blood).

Numbness in Hands
Wash numb or trembling hands in a decoction of wormwood and mustard seed.

Piles
Infuse 1 handful of nettles in 2 pints of water. Strain, and take 1 wineglass of the resulting liquid 2–3 times a day.

Pneumonia
Take 1 handful of white horehound and pulverize finely. Add pure spring water. Allow to stand for 3 hours, then strain through a fine cloth. Add an equal amount of honey. Simmer slowly. Take 1 wineglass every 3 hours.

Rheumatism
Boil 1 oz of celery seed in 1 pint of water. Reduce to ½ pint. Strain, bottle and seal. Take 1 teaspoon twice a day in a little water for 2 weeks.

Hot rum laced with nutmeg and pepper is an old folk cure for rheumatic pains.

Sciatica
Boil 1 handful of nettles until they are soft and mushy. Apply in a cloth as a poultice to the painful area.

Scurvy
Steep 2 oz of dandelion roots and 2 oz of daisies in 6 pints of water. Boil down to 4 pints. Take 1 teacup night and morning.

Senile Decay
An old folk remedy to prevent the onset of senile decay was to boil a handful of nettle leaves and eat them morning and night.

Skin Complaints
For itchy skin, says one eighteenth-century recipe, apply hot water and soap using a corncob. Follow this by a treatment with a mixture of lard and sulphur.

Take 1 handful of coltsfoot flowers and soak them in fresh milk for 3 hours. Remove, and wrap in muslin. Use as a compress to remove unsightly blemishes from the skin.

Mix equal amounts of burdock, yarrow and marshmallow. Soak in boiling water, steep and strain. Drink ½ cup of the resulting liquid 3 times a day, or use as a lotion on the affected part of the skin.

Sores
Mix equal amounts of groundsel, kitchen soap and sugar. Apply to the sore to draw out the infection.

Sore Throats
Pour 1 pint of boiling water on a handful of sage leaves. Infuse for 30 minutes. Add enough vinegar to make it acid to the taste. Sweeten with honey if required. Use as a gargle 3–4 times a day.

Add 1 oz of yarrow root to 1 pint of boiling water. Steep, strain and cool. Take 1 tablespoon 3 times a day.

Add 2 handfuls of elderberries to boiling water and stir well. Put in a little honey to sweeten. Cool, and strain through fine cloth or a kitchen sieve. Sip slowly, as required, to ease the soreness.

An eighteenth-century remedy says mix a pennyworth of camphor in a wineglass of brandy. Pour a small quantity on a lump of loaf sugar. Allow to dissolve in the mouth and repeat every hour. After the fourth dose the sore throat will have gone.

Stings
For relief from insect stings or bites rub crushed marigold leaves on the afflicted part of the body.

Stomach Ache
See Nausea *and* Colic.

Toothache
Mix vinegar, tansy, onion and a few peppercorns. Boil, and carefully strain off the liquid. Place 1 teaspoon of this liquid on the inflamed gum or aching tooth.

Apply a crushed garlic bulb to the gum above tooth – it is alleged to deaden the pain.

Tonic
Mix equal parts of greater yellow gentian root, skullcap, burnet root, betony and spearmint. Soak in boiling water. Strain and cool. Take ½ teaspoon 3 times a day as a tonic to relax the body and calm the mind.

Tuberculosis
Boil 1 lb of honey gently in a saucepan. Finely grate two large sticks of horseradish and stir into the honey. Boil for 5 minutes, stirring well to prevent burning. Transfer into jars to cool. Take 2–3 tablespoons daily.

Ulcers (External)
Grate 2 large carrots and make into a poultice. Apply directly to the ulcer.

Warts
Rub any of the following onto the wart: greater celandine juice, marigold juice, juice of dandelion stems, juice of elder stems, juice of heliotrope leaves mixed with salt, juice of hartstongue fern, fig juice, leek juice, milk thistle juice, St John's wort juice, mullein juice, juice of wheat ears mixed with salt, rue juice, thyme juice boiled in wine with pepper, juice of teazel roots boiled in wine, or the burnt ashes of willow bark mixed with vinegar.

Water Retention
Grind 10 broom seeds into a fine powder and take with honey.

Wounds
Bruise a blackberry leaf and apply to open wounds to stop bleeding.

To aid fast healing, wrap bay leaves soaked in brandy around the wound with a bandage.

Part Three

Practical Folk Medicine

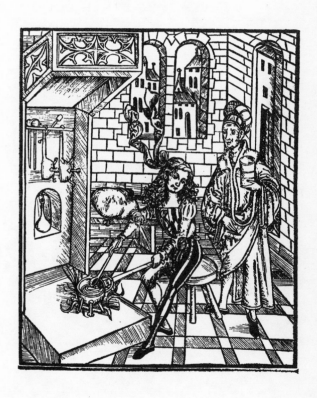

The purpose of this part of the book is to offer the reader practical information on the use of folk remedies, with the emphasis on the identification, preparation and use of common herbs for healing purposes. Different herbs for treating specific medical complaints and diseases are named. As with the folk remedies in Part Two, they have been arranged for easy reference under the diseases and illnesses. Following that is a glossary of medical terms with explanations, which will be of particular use when you come on to Part Four. Practical information is then given on the growing, harvesting and preparation of herbs used in medical remedies.

Herbs of Healing for Specific Diseases and Medical Complaints

Alcoholic Poisoning
Feverfew

Allergies
Eyebright

Anaemia
Angelica
Barberry
Comfrey
Dandelion
Fenugreek
Fumitory
Great yellow gentian
Nettle
St John's wort
Sweet flag
Watercress
Vervain

Appetite, for Improving
Angelica
Buckthorn
Camomile
Caraway
Centaury
Chicory
Coriander
Dandelion
Dill
Great yellow gentian

Horseradish
Lady's mantle
Madder
Marjoram
Mint (peppermint and spearmint)
Mugwort
Parsley
Sorrel
Speedwell
Sweet flag
Tarragon
Thyme
Watercress
Wormwood

Arthritis
Buckthorn
Burdock
Centaury
Chickweed
Comfrey
Elder
Meadowsweet
Restharrow
Violet
Wintergreen
Wormwood

Asthma
Burdock

Butterbur
Camomile
Centaury
Coltsfoot
Comfrey
Garlic
Greater celandine
Horseradish
Lovage
Mullein
Nettle
Parsley
Peony
Thyme
Valerian
Watercress
White horehound

Bed-wetting

Bearberry
Fennel
Hollyhock
Lady's mantle
Mallow
Pansy
Restharrow
St John's wort

Blood Pressure, High

Barberry
Chervil
Comfrey
Garlic
Goose grass
Hawthorn
Onion
Parsley
Rue
Skullcap
Vervain
Violet

Blood Pressure, Low

Broom
Heather
Lavender
Motherwort
Rosemary
Shepherd's purse

Bronchitis

Angelica
Bugle
Butterbur
Caraway
Chervil
Chickweed
Coltsfoot
Comfrey
Daisy
Fennel
Fenugreek
Garlic
Ground Ivy
Hedge Mustard
Houndstongue
Knotgrass
Liquorice
Lungwort
Madder
Mallow
Marjoram
Milkwort
Mouse-ear hawkweed
Mullein
Onion
Parsley
Plantain
Primrose
Savory

Soapwort
Speedwell
Sweet violet
Thyme
Watercress
White horehound

Bruises
Agrimony
Buckthorn
Catnip
Celery
Chickweed
Chicory
Comfrey
Fenugreek
Figwort
Herb Robert
Houndstongue
Mugwort
Primrose
Rosemary
St John's wort
Tansy
White horehound
Wintergreen
Witchhazel

Burns
Burdock
Chickweed
Coltsfoot
Comfrey
Houndstongue
Lady's mantle
Plantain
St John's wort
Witchhazel

Catarrh
See Bronchitis

Chilblains
Angelica
Garlic
Hawthorn
Horseradish
Lady's mantle
Mugwort
Onion
Shepherd's purse
Watercress

Childbirth
Columbine
Comfrey
Flax
Groundsel
Lady's mantle
Pansy
Motherwort
Primrose
Raspberry
White horehound

Colds
Angelica
Avens
Burdock
Catnip
Coltsfoot
Elder
Feverfew
Garlic
Hedge mustard
Horseradish
Lungwort
Maidenhair
Marjoram
Meadowsweet
Onion
Plantain

Rose hip
Sage
Spearmint

Constipation
Asparagus
Buckthorn
Chickweed
Chicory
Dandelion
Elder
Elm
Fat hen
Feverfew
Figwort
Flax
Fumitory
Greater celandine
Groundsel
Hedge mustard
Hollyhock
Horseradish
Lily of the valley
Liquorice
Madder
Mallow
Mugwort
Pansy
Raspberry
Rosehip
Rowan
Soapwort
Sorrel
Strawberry

Coughs
See Bronchitis *and* Colds

Cuts, Sores and Insect Bites
Agrimony

Basil
Betony
Borage
Bugle
Burnet
Butterbur
Camomile
Catnip
Chickweed
Chicory
Coltsfoot
Comfrey
Eyebright
Goose grass
Groundsel
Horsetail
Houndstongue
Kidneywort
Lady's bedstraw
Lady's mantle
Marigold
Marshmallow
Plantain
Purple loosestrife
Raspberry
Sage
St John's wort
Thyme
White horehound
Witchhazel

Cystitis
Angelica
Bearberry
Betony
Comfrey
Couch grass
Fennel
Goose grass
Golden rod

Ground ivy
Lady's mantle
Mallow
Pansy
Parsley piert
Watercress
Yarrow

Diarrhoea
Agrimony
Avens
Cinquefoil
Comfrey
Daisy
Herb Robert
Lungwort
Marjoram
Potentil
Purple loosestrife
Raspberry
Sage
Slippery elm
Sorrel

Eye Disorders
Angelica
Borage
Cornflower
Eyebright
Fumitory
Herb Robert
Marigold
Meadowsweet

Fever
Angelica
Betony
Borage
Catnip
Cowslip

Feverfew
Lilac
Limeflowers
Lovage
Meadowsweet
Pink
Poppy
Sage
Viper's bugloss
White horehound
Yarrow

Flatulence
Angelica
Caraway
Catnip
Celery
Coriander
Dill
Fennel
Feverfew
Horseradish
Lavender
Peppermint
Spearmint
Sweet flag
Tansy
Tarragon
Woodruff
See also Indigestion

Gall Bladder Disorders
Betony
Marigold
Peony
Pimpernel
Purple flag
Vervain

Gallstones and Kidney Stones
Barberry
Chicory

Knotgrass
Madder
Parsley piert
Restharrow

Gums, Sore, and Mouth Ulcers
Avens
Cinquefoil
Columbine
Comfrey
Herb Robert
Hollyhock
Marshmallow
Periwinkle
Raspberry
Savory
Self heal
Vervain

Halitosis
Avens
Dill
Peppermint

Headache and Migraine
Angelica
Basil
Betony
Feverfew
Lavender
Limeflowers
Pennyroyal
Peppermint
Primrose
Spearmint
St John's wort
Valerian
Viper's bugloss
Wintergreen

Heart Trouble
Broom
Bugle
Burnet
Figwort
Gipsywort
Great yellow gentian
Hawthorn
Hedge mustard
Lily of the valley
Motherwort
Raspberry
Viper's bugloss
Woodruff

Haemorrhoids
See Piles

Hysteria
Betony
Catnip
Centaury
Lady's bedstraw
Lavender
Lily of the valley
Peppermint
Motherwort
Poppy
Skullcap
St John's wort
Sweet flag
Valerian
Vervain
Viper's bugloss
Watercress

Indigestion
Dill
Fennel
Feverfew

Mugwort
Peppermint
Spearmint
Speedwell
Thyme
See also Flatulence

Influenza
See Colds

Insect Bites
See Cuts.

Insomnia
Catnip
Camomile
Dandelion
Dill
Hawthorn
Heather
Peppermint
Poppy
Primrose
Skullcap
Valerian
Woodruff

Kidney Disorders
Agrimony
Angelica
Bearberry
Betony
Broom
Daisy
Dandelion
Fumitory
Golden rod
Heather
Horsetail
Kidneywort

Parsley
Peony
Restharrow
Shepherd's purse
Strawberry

Kidney Stones
See Gallstones

Lactation, for Improving
Basil
Borage
Caraway
Dill
Fennel
Milkwort
Motherwort
Raspberry

Liver Disorders
Agrimony
Avens
Daisy
Mouse-ear hawkweed
Purple flag
Rosemary

Lung Disease
Comfrey
Knotgrass
Lungwort
Primrose

Menstruation, Inhibited
Marigold
Motherwort
Mugwort
Rue
Shepherd's purse
Southernwood

Tarragon

Menstruation, Excessive
Broom
Bugle
Burnet
Marigold
Moneywort
Mugwort
Periwinkle
Rue
Yarrow

Migraine
See Headache

Mouth Ulcers
See Gums

Nervous Disorders
See Hysteria

Period Pains
Groundsel
Lavender
Motherwort
Pennyroyal
Potentil
Rue
Skullcap

Piles
Figwort
Ground ivy
Horse chestnut
Peony
Pilewort
Potentil
Vervain

Rheumatism
Angelica
Asparagus
Burdock
Celery
Chickweed
Coriander
Daisy
Golden rod
Lilac
Meadow saffron
Meadowsweet
Nettle
St John's wort
Wintergreen

Sciatica
Broom
Ground elder
Ground ivy
Kidneywort
St John's wort
Wintergreen

Sinus Troubles
See Bronchitis

Skin Complaints
Avens
Betony
Borage
Burdock
Burnet
Butterbur
Camomile
Catnip
Chervil
Chickweed
Coltsfoot
Comfrey

Fenugreek
Figwort
Flax
Goose grass
Greater celandine
Groundsel
Heather
Herb Robert
Kidneywort
Lady's bedstraw
Lady's mantle
Lavender
Limeflowers
Madder
Nettle
Pansy
Peppermint
Primrose
Purple flag
Raspberry
Restharrow
Rosemary
Slippery elm
Soapwort
Sorrel
Speedwell
Tansy
White horehound
Witchhazel

Sore Throats
Agrimony
Avens
Caraway
Columbine
Comfrey
Fennel
Fenugreek
Figwort
Ground ivy

Hedge mustard
Herb Robert
Lovage
Lungwort
Mallow
Periwinkle
Plantain
Potentil
Purple loosestrife
Rowan
Sage
Savory
Self heal
Wintergreen

Sores
See Cuts

Stomach Complaints
Angelica
Basil
Caraway
Centaury
Chicory
Cinquefoil
Comfrey
Fennel
Feverfew
Garlic
Great yellow gentian
Greater celandine
Groundsel
Horsetail
Houndstongue
Kidneywort
Knotgrass
Lady's smock
Mallow
Marigold
Marjoram

Marshmallow
Meadowsweet
Milkwort
Moneywort
Rue
Slippery elm
Speedwell
Sweet flag
Tarragon

Toothache
Broom
Clove
Lavender
Marjoram
Wintergreen

Ulcers, Mouth,
See Gums

Water Retention
Agrimony
Asparagus
Bearberry

Broom
Buckthorn
Chervil
Dandelion
Golden rod
Heather
Hedge mustard
Kidneywort
Lady's smock
Lily of the valley
Madder
Maidenhair
Onion
Pansy
Pimpernel
Plantain
Restharrow
Rowan
Shepherd's purse
Sorrel
Speedwell
Watercress
Yarrow

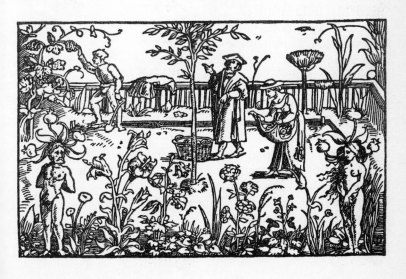

Common Medical Terms

The following terms, used to describe the healing properties of various herbs, are in common use among qualified medical herbalists and practitioners of folk medicine.

Anaesthetic   agent which produces insensibility to pain.
Alterative   agent causing alterations in medical conditions.
Analgesic   agent which deadens pain.
Anthelmintic   agent which expels worms.
Antibiotic   destroys bacteria.
Anticoagulant   prevents blood clotting.
Antiemetic   relieves vomiting.
Antilithic   dissolves gall or kidney stones.
Antiphlogistic   reduces inflammation.
Antipyretic   reduces fever.
Antiseptic   reduces or destroys harmful bacteria.
Antispasmodic   relieves muscular spasms and cramps.
Aperient   mild laxative.
Appetizer   promotes appetite.
Aphrodisiac   stimulates sexual desire.
Asthmatic   agent used to treat asthma.
Astringent   reduces secretions or discharges.
Calmative   mild sedative with calming effect.
Cardiac   stimulates heart.
Carminative   expels stomach gases from intestines.
Cathartic   laxative.
Coagulant   clots blood.
Cholagogue   agent that increases flow of bile to intestines.
Demulcent   soothes irritation.
Depressant   reduces nervousness.
Depurative   purifies blood.
Digestive   promotes digestion.
Diuretic   promotes urinary flow.

Emmenagogue promotes menstrual flow.

Emollient softens hard tissues.

Expectorant promotes discharge of mucus from respiratory passages.

Febrifuge agent which dispels fever.

Galactagogue increases secretion of breast milk.

Hydragogue agent which expels water from the body.

Hydrotic agent which promotes perspiration.

Laxative promotes bowel movement.

Narcotic agent which induces sleep or loss of consciousness.

Nervine calms nerves.

Stomachic stimulates stomach.

Tonic promotes good health and energy.

Vermifuge agent which expels worms and other parasites from intestines.

Vulnerary heals wounds.

Preparation of Herbs for Healing

Growing, Drying and Storage

Although herbs can be bought from commercial herb gardens and herb suppliers, if you are to become seriously involved in folk medicine you are recommended to attempt to grow your own raw materials. Herbs are comparatively easy to cultivate. Most of them are hardy plants which do not take up much room in the garden and, once well established, need very little attention. Although herbs usually grow in profusion in the wild, some care is required in first establishing them. The garden should be well drained, and preferably in a sunny, sheltered spot.

One essential requirement for the successful cultivation of herbs is fertile soil. Organic compost or fertilizer can be used, but herbs do not respond well to chemically based fertilizers or pesticides. Nor do they like a soil which is poorly balanced in minerals, and if your projected herb garden has that kind of soil it will need considerable attention before you begin planting.

As you will be growing your herbs not for decorative purposes but for use in medical remedies, arrange your garden so that the plants can be harvested easily. Make a plan of the area you will be using to grow the herbs, so that different kinds of plants can be grown in clumps. A formal herb garden of this type does not need a lot of ground – you will be amazed at how many different varieties of healing plants can be cultivated in a small area. Once the herb garden is established keep weeds under control so that the plants remain healthy.

Harvesting the herbs before using them in folk remedies is a subject which the old herbalists spend many pages of their textbooks describing. We need not go into such detail, but a few simple rules should still be followed. The old herbals recommended that the blossoms and leaves should be collected in spring and early summer; the fruits and berries would be gathered in late summer or early autumn, while the seeds were to be harvested in late autumn or early winter. This sequence of harvesting follows the natural cycle of the seasons and is quite logical. Obviously you pick only those plants which look healthy and disease-free. The ideal time to gather herbs which are not for immediate use and are to be dried and stored is on a sunny morning when the dew has evaporated from the grass. Handle the herbs as carefully as possible so as not to break the stems or bruise the leaves, and take them indoors immediately after picking.

To dry herbs, hang them from the ceiling in small bunches in a dark place. Alternatively lay them out on wooden racks covered with gauze or sheets of white paper. Although the place in which you dry the herbs must be warm, there should also be a free flow of air to prevent must forming on the plants, or premature rotting. Professional herbalists sometimes speed up the drying process by exposing the plants to artificial sources of heat. At home, either use a well ventilated airing cupboard, or put the herbs near a kitchen range such as a Rayburn or Aga. Never expose herbs to direct heat for drying.

Once the herbs have been dried they can be stored in airtight glass containers in a dark cupboard away from direct light. Alternatively they can be stored in plastic bags, although for obvious reasons this can create condensation problems. Remember to label each container with the herb it contains and the date it was harvested.

Making Up Herbal Remedies

Preparing the herbal remedy correctly is one of the most important aspects of the practice of folk medicine. Herbs for healing purposes can be applied in several different ways: ointments, salves and poultices for external use, and infusions and decoctions for internal use. The leaves and flowers of herbs can be soaked in water to distil their essence, but roots and seeds will have to be crushed or powdered. Herbal remedies are best made from fresh ingredients, and if possible they should be used within twelve hours of collection. If medicinal herbs are to be stored longer they should certainly be used within twelve months of harvesting. Seeds and roots can be kept for several years before they become no longer potent enough to work effective cures. Under normal circumstances, especially if you have a herb garden, you will be using fresh raw materials each season and will only need to store a back-up supply for the winter months.

Infusion is the most popular form of utilizing the healing power of herbs where only the leaves, stems and flowers are to be used. A simple process, it involves soaking the herbs in boiling water to create a beverage. The herbs should be boiled in a china, stone or heatproof glass vessel fitted with a tight lid, which helps to prevent the escape of volatile ingredients released from the herbs during distillation. Alternatively, boiling water can be poured over the herbs in the vessel as if you were making tea.

The usual quantity of herbal raw materials used in this distillation method is approximately ½–1 oz added to a pint of boiling water, although exact quantities vary from one herbalist to the next. For best results herbs should be infused for 10–15 minutes. The infused liquid is then strained through a piece of muslin or a fine kitchen sieve into a cup or glass and allowed to cool. If a bitter-tasting herb has been used, a small quantity of brown sugar or honey can be added as a natural sweetener.

The second method used by folk healers and herbalists to prepare herbs for medicinal purposes is called **decoction**; it is suitable for bark, roots and seeds. Approximately 1 oz of herbal raw material is added to 20 fl. oz of cold water in an enamel or glass container and allowed to soak for 10–15 minutes. The temperature is then raised to boiling point and the mixture simmered for 10–15 minutes, after which it is allowed to cool for another 10 minutes. During both processes the container in which the herbal mixture has been placed should be covered. Once the decoction is completed the liquid is strained through a fine cloth or sieve.

The final popular method for using herbs is poultices and ointments. To make a **poultice** you use herbs which have been freshly gathered, bruised and then crushed to a pulp using a pestle and mortar. The resulting pulped material is then mixed with a quantity of hot water. Alternatively dried herbs can be used as a base, and softened by adding cornmeal or flour. When applying the poultice to the patient put the herbal mixture between thin layers of cloth and then apply it direct to the afflicted part of the body.

The simplest method of making **ointments** is to mix 1 part of the powdered plant with 4 parts of lard or vegetable fat. Alternatively the herbs can be distilled, as in the infusion process, and the resulting liquid added to olive oil or any vegetable fat or oil. Add a small quantity of the dried herb left over from the distillation to provide a firm base for the ointment.

A basic **herbal syrup** can be made by dissolving 3 lb of brown sugar in 1 pint of boiling water. Boil the water again until a thick, syrupy substance is created, and then add the herbs.

Herbal teas can be made by infusing approximately 2–3 teaspoons of dried or freshly picked herbs in 1 pint of boiling water. Leave to brew for a few minutes. Always use a pottery or china teapot, never a metal one.

Dried herbs can be powdered using a pestle and mortar and taken in small quantities sprinkled on food or in water, milk or soup. They can also be mixed in hot or cold water, using a ratio of approximately 1 teaspoon to a ¼ glass of water.

Part Four

A Herbal Glossary

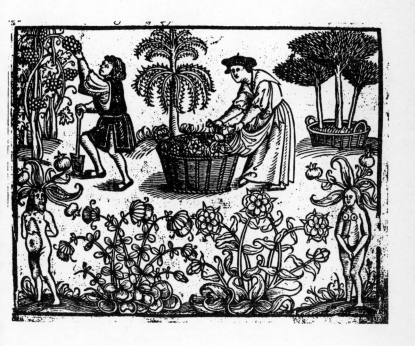

What follows is a glossary of the most common herbs in the British Isles which are used for healing in folk medicine. It covers botanical, medical and folklore aspects of herbalism as well as the application of the herbs in remedies. The information is presented in the following sequence for easy reference:

Botanical name
Popular name(s)
Habitat
Flora and general information
Folklore
General medical properties
Specific properties
Application and use

Healing plants with a high toxicity, such as deadly nightshade, have been excluded from the glossary. Although such plants have a long tradition of use in folk medicine they are generally regarded as too poisonous for use by nonprofessionals. Other plants have toxic capabilities, but can be used under restriction or in small quantities. These plants have been included in the glossary, but with the proviso that they are only used under the direction of a qualified medical herbalist. The majority of herbs are safe in use, but obviously common sense needs to be used in dealing with any botanically derived raw material which is used for medical purposes. If you find you are suffering an unpleasant reaction to any plant material consult a medical herbalist.

AGRIMONY

Botanical name: *Agrimonia eupatoria*.

Popular names: Church steeples, sticklewort.

Habitat: Hedge banks, copses and field borders.

Flora: Perennial, with small yellow flowers July–August.

Folklore: The name agrimony is derived from the Green *argemone*, meaning 'a white speck in the eye'. According to Nicholas Culpeper, this herb was sacred to the planet Jupiter and was ruled astrologically by the zodiac sign of Cancer (21 June to 20 July). Pliny the Elder described agrimony as a 'herb of sovereign power'. In the medieval period agrimony was said to possess magical powers, and was specially recommended as a cure for insomnia. It was said by the old herbalists that if agrimony 'be leyd under a mann's hede he shalt sleep as if he were dede. He shat never waken till from under his hede it be taken.' For this reason the herb was a popular ingredient in herbal pillows. Agrimony was included in a fifteenth-century folk remedy to heal musket wounds, and was also reputed to be able to ward off witchcraft. Its popular folk name of church steeples is derived from the shape of its tall flower spikes. Writing about the medicinal qualities of the plant, Gerard said that the leaves of agrimony are 'good for them that have naughty livers'.

General medical properties: Astringent, tonic, diuretic and expectorant.

Specific properties: This herb has a beneficial effect on the liver, kidneys and bladder. It promotes the flow of urine, prevents diarrhoea, can be used as an expectorant for persistent coughs and as a herbal gargle for sore throats. It should be used with caution for constipation, and can be applied externally on wounds or skin complaints such as acne. A poultice made from the herb will treat insect bites and stings. In the old days agrimony was believed to have the ability to draw out splinters from the flesh.

Application and use: Infuse the herb by pouring approximately ¼ pint of boiling water onto ½ teaspoon of dried agrimony. Leave for 15 minutes and then take 3 times daily.

ANGELICA

Botanical name: *Angelica archangelica.*

Popular names: Holy Ghost, archangel, masterwort.

Habitat: River Banks, damp fields and meadows.

Flora: Biennial or perennial, with greenish-white flowers May–August.

Folklore: Angelica derives its religious-sounding name from the fact that it is usually in flower on the Christian festival of St Michael on 8 May. Despite these orthodox religious associations, angelica was a plant widely prized by the pagans. With the coming of the new religion its pagan overtones were reversed, and it became a magical plant which had the power to protect its user from the powers of darkness. This was because in Hebrew mythology St Michael was the guardian of the gates of the underworld and waged war against the rebel archangel Lucifer. In the Middle Ages it is recorded that angelica grew freely in many London fields; it was collected by the old herbalists and folk healers as it had many medicinal and culinary uses. Because of its fragrance, angelica was widely used in crystallized form as a cake decoration. Its seeds are used in the making of vermouth. In his famous *Herbal*, Gerard states that the flowers of angelica baked with sugar or distilled water extracted from them 'makes the heart merry' and 'makes good the colour of the face and refreshes the vital spirits'. During the Great Plague of 1665 Londoners chewed pieces of angelica root in the belief that it would save them from catching the disease.

General medical properties: Appetizer, carminative, expectorant, stimulant, stomachic, tonic and diuretic.

Specific properties: Angelica will stimulate the appetite after long illnesses and is also recommended in cases of anorexia nervosa. It is used for treating anaemia, migraine, vertigo and general dizziness for whatever cause. The candied roots can be eaten to ward off infection and warm the stomach. As an expectorant the herb helps coughs, influenza, colds, sore throats and bronchitis. It helps to calm fevers, and eases flatulence and indigestion. Angelica can also be used to cure cystitis and as a urinary antiseptic. Good results have been achieved with this herb for treating muscular cramps, stimulating kidney action, and preventing nervous headaches and rheumatic pain. Angelica tea is good for improving bad eyesight and relieving deafness. Externally the plant can be used for chilblains.

Application and use: Infuse 1 teaspoon of crushed seeds in ½ cup of boiling water. Take 1 cup before each meal.

ASPARAGUS

Botanical name: *Asparagus officinalis*.

Popular names: Garden asparagus, sparrow grass.

Habitat: Cultivated.
Flora: Perennial, with whitish-green flowers in May and June.

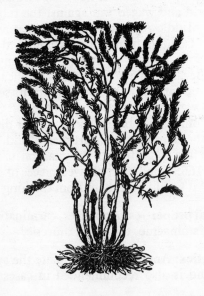

Folklore: The name of this plant is derived from a Greek word which means 'to sprout', referring to the fleshy shoots which are used in cookery. This plant has been cultivated for over two thousand years. It was used by the old herbalists both as a cure for constipation and for its alleged power to revive the sexual abilities of the impotent!

General medical properties: Diuretic and laxative.

Specific properties: Asparagus is recommended for the treatment of kidney disorders, water retention, gout and rheumatic pains.

Application and use: Infuse 1 teaspoon of the root stock in 1 cup of boiling water for 15 minutes. Take 1 cup a day.

AVENS

Botanical name: *Geum urbanum.*

Popular names: Colewort, herb bennet, St Benedict's herb.

Habitat: Woodland, hedgerows and ditches.

Flora: Perennial, with yellow flowers May – July.

Folklore: This plant gained its popular name of St Benedict's herb from the medieval *herba benedicta*, meaning the blessed herb. Because of its strong aromatic properties it allegedly had the magical power to drive away evil spirits. It was also believed that anyone who carried a sprig of this herb would not be bitten by rabid dogs or poisonous snakes. The leaves grow in threes, so the herb became associated with the Holy Trinity of the Father, Son and Holy Ghost; in addition, in Christian flower lore its five-petalled flowers symbolized the wounds suffered by Jesus on the cross. According to Culpeper, this plant was governed by the planet Jupiter; both he and Gerard recommended its use as an antidote to poison and animal bites. Paracelsus suggested that avens should be used to treat catarrh, stomach upsets and liver disease. In folk belief it was said that if you dug up the root of this plant before sunrise and hung it in a linen bag around your neck it would cure piles and strengthen the eyesight.

General medical properties: Astringent, stomachic and cardiac.

Specific properties: Avens is recommended for the cure of diarrhoea; it prevents vomiting and catarrh and can be used to ease the symptoms of the common cold. It can also be prescribed for heart disease, obstructions of the liver and the prevention of colic. It is used as a throat gargle and for the treatment of halitosis and mouth ulcers. Externally, it removes spots and blemishes from the skin.

Application and use: Boil 1 teaspoon of the root in ¼ pint of water and simmer for 5–10 minutes. Take 1 cup a day.

BALM

Botanical name: *Melissa officinalis.*

Popular names: Garden balm, sweet balm, lemon balm.

Habitat:
Cultivated, or on roadsides and in hedgerows.

Flora:
Perennial, with yellowish-white flowers in July.

Folklore:
This plant has the fragrance of lemons, hence its folk name of lemon balm. Its name in fact derives from a Greek word meaning 'bee', because large numbers of bees are attracted to the flowers. In southern Europe, where the plant originated, it is widely used for culinary purposes to flavour soups and salads.

General medical properties: Stimulant and carminative.

Specific properties: Balm is recommended for treating headaches, coughs and influenza, and for breaking fevers.

Application and use: Infuse 1–2 teaspoon of the dried herb in 1 cup of boiling water. Take one cup daily.

BARBERRY

Botanical name: *Berberis vulgaris.*

Popular names: Common barberry, sow berry.

Habitat: Woodland and hedgerows.

Flora: Perennial shrub, with yellow flowers May–June.

Folklore: This medicinal plant with its distinctive purple berries is much loved by pigs, hence one of its common names. It was introduced into Europe by medieval monks who cultivated it in their gardens; they ate the ripe fruits as a preserve and used the yellow dye which can be extracted from the roots for dyeing cloth. In ancient Egypt the barberry was used with fennel seeds as a cure for plague. The old herbals recommended the use of this plant as a gargle for sore throats and as a purgative for which it is renowned. Barberry is becoming rarer, as it is the host plant of the black rust fungi which attacks wheat, and for this reason is regarded as an enemy by farmers.

General medical properties: Cholagogue and astringent.

Specific properties: Barberry contains an alkaloid known as berberine which has astringent qualities. It is recommended as a mouthwash and throat gargle, also for use in remedies for curing dysentery, lowering blood pressure, dissolving kidney stones and as a purgative. The herb is also useful in cases of vitamin C deficiency as it has a high content of that vitamin.

Application and use: Infuse 1 teaspoon of the plant in 1 cup of boiling water. Infuse for 15 minutes. Take 1 cup daily.

BASIL

Botanical name: *Ocimum basilicum*.

Popular names: Sweet basil, garden basil, St Joseph's wort.

Habitat: Cultivated as culinary herb.

Flora: Perennial, with white to red flowers blooming June–September.

Folklore: Basil has been grown for centuries in kitchen gardens for use in cooking, and is recommended for use in sauces, dressings, soups and as a garnish. The herb is believed to have been introduced into the British Isles from Asia as late as the sixteenth century. In India it is recorded that basil was regarded as the sacred herb of the pantheon of Hindu gods and goddesses. To the ancient Cretans and Romans it was a symbol of love, a tradition which survived in popular English folklore – country people said that anyone who grew basil in their garden would never be short of admirers of the opposite sex. In the Middle Ages basil was used to alleviate the labour pains of expectant mothers and was said to be able to draw out the poison of scorpion stings. The latter attribute may come from the similarity of the Latin *Basilicum* to *Basilisk*, a mythical reptile hatched by a serpent from a hen's egg; anyone who came under the gaze of this creature was immediately struck down dead. In fact the common name of the herb is an abbreviation of the Greek *basilikon phuton*, meaning 'kingly herb'. Because of its strong smell basil was often used as a room freshener in medieval times.

General medical properties: Mild sedative, antispasmodic, digestive, appetizer, carminative and galactagogue.

Specific properties: Basil is recommended as a sedative, for stopping stomach cramps, vomiting, constipation and headaches, and in the treatment of whooping cough. It also helps relieve insomnia, migraine, dizziness and vertigo. The soothing oil of basil is recommended for treating insect stings, bites and minor scratches or cuts. Finally, the herb is reputed to be able to increase the flow of breast milk in nursing mothers.

Application and use: Infuse 1 teaspoon of the dried herb in ¼ pint of boiling water. Take 1 tablespoon 3 times a day. Mixed with sage it makes an excellent herbal tea.

BEARBERRY

Botanical name: *Arctostaphylos uva-ursi.*

Popular names: Bear's grape, whortberry, mountain box, red box.

Habitat: Woodland, heathland and hills.

Flora: Evergreen shrub, with white or pink flowers May–June.

Folklore: The scientific and popular names of this plant originate in the Greek *arkton staphyle* meaning 'bear's grapes'; in past times the glossy red berries of the shrub were regarded as a delicacy by the native European bear. The plant was used by rural folk healers in thirteenth-century Wales as an antiseptic but was not officially recognized until the eighteenth century.

General medical properties: Diuretic and antiseptic.

Specific properties: The active ingredients of bearberry leaves are hydroquionone and arbutin, both of which have an astringent effect which is useful for treating inflamed urinary tracts, especially in cystitis. A harmless side-effect of its use is that the patient's urine turns bright green. The leaves also contain a substance called allantoin which soothes and heals irritated body tissue. Today, bearberry is used principally for kidney disorders and water retention.

Application and use: Infuse 1 teaspoon of dried leaves in 1 cup of hot water. Cool, and take 2–3 cups a day. *Over-use can cause constipation.*

BETONY

Botanical name: *Stachys officinalis.*

Popular names: Wood betony, lousewort, common betony.

Habitat: Woodland and meadows.

Flora: Perennial, with reddish-purple flowers June–August.

Folklore: Allegedly the common name of this herb derives from an old Celtic word *bewton,* meaning 'good for the head', but this may be only speculative. Betony does have a long history as a magical plant with occult powers. Antonius Musa, physician to the Roman Emperor Augustus Caesar, wrote a book on the virtues of this herb, claiming that it was a good protection against evil and sorcery. An old superstition claimed that if two snakes were placed within a ring of betony they would fight to the death; possibly because of this belief the herb was regarded as a cure for snakebites and attacks by rabid dogs. In the old days betony was planted in churchyards, allegedly to stop the spirits of the dead from walking at night. If gathered without the use of an iron implement, betony was said to cure drunkenness. In his *Herbal* Culpeper assigned this herb to the rulership of the planet Jupiter and the zodiac sign of Aries, the ram (21 March–20 April).

General medical properties: Nervine, sedative, tonic, expectorant and asthmatic.

Specific properties: Betony is recommended for treating gallstones, heartburn and high blood pressure. It also prevents excessive sweating and the spitting of blood. Because it works on the central nervous system it is ideal for treating migraine, nervousness and neuralgia. It also acts as a mild sedative and tonic and is recommended for treating kidney infections. Externally, it can be used in an ointment for the treatment of boils, sores and cuts.

Application and use: Infuse ½ teaspoon in 1 cup of boiling water. Take once or twice a day.

BLACKBERRY

Botanical name: *Rubus fruticosus*.

Popular name: Bramble.

Habitat: Hedgerows and cultivated.

Flora: Shrub, with whitish-pink flowers June–September. Blackish-red berries September–October.

Folklore: The common name, bramble, is derived from the word *brom*, meaning 'thorny shrub'. In Germany the plant is still known as *Brombeere*. Culpeper assigned this plant to the ancient goddess of love, Venus; he also said, however, that it was ruled by the astrological sign of Aries, which comes under Mars – this was because the shrub has soft fruit but prickly thorns. Gerard recommended that blackberry leaves should be boiled in water with honey and white wine as a mouthwash for gum ulcers or as a lotion for sores on 'the privie parts'.

General medical properties: Astringent, tonic and diuretic.

Specific properties: Blackberry is recommended as a gargle for sore throats, for water retention and as a general tonic. The berries are rich in vitamin C and therefore good for preventing colds and influenza.

Application and use: Infuse 1 handful of berries in 1 pint of hot water. Take as a gargle for a sore throat or drink as a general tonic.

BORAGE

Botanical name: *Borago officinalis*.

Popular names: Bugloss, cool tankard, burrage.

Habitat: Culinary herb cultivated in gardens but also found wild.

Flora: Annual, with blue-purple star-shaped flowers June–August.

Folklore: Borage is a well-known cultivated herb widely used in cordials and cooling drinks. The name borage is said to derive from Arabic *abou rach*, meaning 'father of all sweat', a reference to the herb's alleged properties of promoting perspiration, for which reason it was recommended for treating fevers. The ancients believed that borage could cure melancholy by creating a state of euphoria: if drunk in moderate quantities, an infusion of borage allegedly had the effect of lowering the inhibitions and made the drinker talk profusely. Because the herb attracts bees it was always planted near hives. Its candied flowers were used for cake decorations, and its roots for flavouring wine.

General medical properties: Demulcent, diuretic, hydrotic and stimulant.

Specific properties: Borage promotes the flow of urine and perspiration and can therefore be used to treat fevers, chills and influenza. Externally, it can be made into a poultice for cooling inflammation.

Application and use: Infuse 1 teaspoon of fresh flowers or 2–3 teaspoons of dried flowers with ½ cup of water. Steep for 5 minutes and then strain. Alternatively, fresh borage leaves can be crushed with watercress or dandelion leaves to make a herbal juice.

BROOM

Botanical name: *Cytisus scoparius*.

Popular names: Common broom, he broom (without flowers), she broom (with flowers).

Habitat: Heathland, woodland and sandy places.

Flora: Perennial, with yellow flowers throughout summer.

Folklore: Traditionally, in popular folklore this plant has a sinister image. According to an old rhyme which originates in Sussex,

> If you sweep the house with blossomed broom in May
> You will sweep the head of the household away.

Despite this grim warning, country weddings always featured a bundle of green broom tied with multi-coloured ribbons as a good luck charm. Broom has always been associated with witchcraft. In heraldry it was the plant of the Plantagenet kings, who some historians believe may have been the secret leaders of the medieval witch cult. Their family name of Plantagenet is derived from one of the Latin names for broom, *Planta genista*. Medieval herbalists mixed the burnt ashes of broom with white wine to cure dropsy (water retention). Its pungent smell was said to have the power to calm wild horses and rabid dogs. It has a very strong, unpleasant taste.

General medical properties: Cardiac, diuretic, emetic and anticoagulant.

Specific properties: Broom is used to treat heart disease and kidney disorders and to increase urinary flow. It also treats low blood pressure and reduces excessive menstrual flow. It has been used to cure toothache, sciatica and gout. *Use with caution.*

Application and use: *Only under the direction of a medical herbalist.*

BRYONY
See White Bryony.

BUCKTHORN

Botanical name: *Rhamnus catharticus.*

Popular names: Purging buckthorn, waythorn, hart's horn, herb ivy, wortcress, black alder, alder buckthorn.

Habitat: Woodland and hedgerows.

Flora: Perennial, with greenish flowers May–June. Black berries ripen in September.

Folklore: Buckthorn, first recorded in Anglo-Saxon times, is renowned in folk medicine for its purgative qualities. Its straight, flexible branches are used to make wickerwork furniture. The pigment known as sap green is derived from the juice of the berries mixed with limewater and gum arabic. The woody parts were used in the old days to produce a charcoal that was employed in the manufacture of gunpowder.

General medical properties: Laxative and diuretic.

Specific properties: The general use of buckthorn in folk remedies is as a purgative to relieve constipation and increase urine flow in cases of water retention. Externally, it can be used to treat bruises.

Application and use: Infuse 1 teaspoon of *matured* dried bark in 1½ pints of boiling water in a covered container for approximately 30 minutes. Cool, and take 1 tablespoon morning and evening. *Use with caution. Do not use fresh bark and do not overdose, which produces vomiting and stomach pains as side-effects. If in any doubt about its use consult a medical herbalist.*

BUGLE

Botanical name: *Ajuga reptans.*

Popular names: Common bugle, creeping bugle, carpenter's bugle, bugle weed.

Habitat: Woodland and fields.

Flora: Perennial, with white or pink flowers May–July.

Folklore: One of the common names, carpenter's herb, indicates its use in folk medicine – it was said to be able to stem the flow of blood from cuts. As well as preventing bleeding, bugle contains an unknown ingredient, similiar to digitalis, which acts as a heart tonic.

General medical properties: Astringent, cardiac stimulant, expectorant and anti-haemorrhagic.

Specific properties: Principally used as an agent to stop bleeding from open wounds. Also inhibits menstrual flow, relieves bronchitis and acts as a tonic for the heart.

Application and use: Infuse 1 teaspoon of the herb in a cup of boiling water for 15 minutes. Take 1 cup a day.

BURDOCK

Botanical name: *Arctium lappa*.

Popular names: Cockle buttons, cat's bur, gypsy rhubarb, beggar's buttons, thorny burr.

Habitat: Ditches, watersides, hedges and wasteland.

Flora: Biennial, with purple flowers July–September.

Folklore: Burdock is popular with children because of its tiny burs, which cling to clothes; it is mentioned in Shakespeare's play *King Lear* on this account. In various parts of Europe and the Far East this herb is actively cultivated for culinary purposes: its young leaves are eaten in salads and the root can be boiled and served with butter to make a pleasant vegetable. It resembles rhubarb, hence one of its popular names which indicates that it was highly regarded by gypsies. Gerard said that the juice of the burdock leaf mixed with honey 'procureth urine and taketh away the pains of the bladder'.

General medical properties: Alterative, diuretic and tonic.

Specific properties: Burdock is recommended externally to treat skin complaints including boils, eczema and psoriasis. It is also said to be useful in the treatment of arthritis, rheumatic pains, bronchitis and asthma. It is an excellent blood purifier and can be used to heal burns.

Application and use: Infuse 3 teaspoons of finely chopped leaves in 1 pint of boiling water for 10 minutes. For bruises or external inflammation, apply a poultice of fresh leaves boiled for 5 minutes in lightly salted water. A hair lotion to prevent premature baldness can be made up by macerating 4 oz of fresh root and 2 oz of fresh nettle root for 8 days in a pint of rum. Massage the scalp daily with this mixture.

BURNET

Botanical name: *Sanguisorba officinalis.*

Popular name: Meadow pimpernel.

Habitat: Cultivated in gardens and growing wild in dry, grassy places.

Flora: Perennial, with purple flowers June–July.

Folklore: According to Culpeper, this plant used to grow wild in the fields next to St Pancras church in London and by a causeway in a field near Piccadilly. He assigned burnet astrologically to the sun, and described it as a 'precious herb', claiming that its frequent use 'preserves the body in health and the spirit in vigour'.

General medical properties: Tonic, astringent, cardiac and vulnerary.

Specific properties: Burnet is generally used as a tonic. It is also recommended for heart disease, for inhibiting menstrual flow and for healing open wounds and running sores.

Application and use: Burnet can be made into an ointment for external use, and the leaves can be infused for internal use.

BUTTERBUR

Botanical name: *Petasites hybridus.*

Popular names: Bog rhubarb, devil's hat.

Habitat: Wet places near rivers and ditches.

Flora: Perennial, with blue or red flowers in February–March.

Folklore: The botanical name is derived from the Greek *petasos*, a large hat – a reference to the shape and size of the leaves. The French herbalists called it devil's hat, but the reason is obscure. Its commonest name may derive from the fact that butter was once wrapped in its leaves. Culpeper described butterbur as 'a great preserver of the heart and cheerer of the vital spirits'. He also recommended its use to promote perspiration, for which reason it was used to treat the bubonic plague in the Middle Ages, and suggested that 'it were well if gentlewomen would keep this root preserved to help their poor neighbours' for 'it is fit the rich should help the poor for the poor cannot help themselves'. Among butterbur's other attributes was the power to kill tapeworms, a common problem in the days when inadequate hygiene was combined with a poor diet.

General medical properties: Antispasmodic, expectorant, astringent, febrifuge, vulnerary and diueretic.

Specific properties: Butterbur has a great many uses in folk medicine – for treating coughs, reducing fever, healing open wounds, curing stammering, and relieving stomach cramps and period pains. Because it is a muscle relaxant it can be recommended for general stress, headaches and asthma. Externally, as well as healing open wounds and cuts it can be applied as a poultice, using the leaves to reduce the swelling in bruises and to treat skin diseases. It is also used in cases of water retention as a diuretic.

Application and use: Infuse 1 teaspoon of the root in 1 cup of boiling water. Simmer for 15 minutes. Cool, and drink 1 cup of the infused liquid 3 times a day.

CAMOMILE

Botanical name: *Anthemis nobilis*.

Popular name: Chamomile.

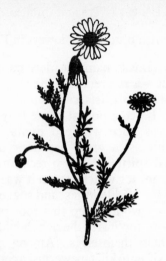

Habitat: Cultivated and wild, in grass and heathland.

Flora: Perennial, with yellow-white flowers June–July.

Folklore: The use of this herb dates back to ancient Egypt, and camomile lotion is still widely used for treating skin disorders. In the Middle Ages herbalists used camomile flowers soaked in white wine as a cure for dropsy (water retention) and jaundice. In the past, because of its ground-covering ability, this plant was used to create lawns, hence the old saying: 'A camomile bed, the more it is trod the more it will spread.' Camomile was also very popular in cottage gardens because it was believed to have the almost mystical power of reviving wilting plants next to it. For cosmetic purposes, essence of camomile was used as a skin cleanser, and a dye was made from the flowers to lighten the hair.

General medical properties: Antispasmodic, sedative, appetizer, diuretic and demulcent.

Specific properties: Camomile is recommended for the treatment of fevers, insomnia and joint pains, for increasing appetite after long illnesses, for relieving period pains, for controlling bad coughs (as an antispasmodic) and for asthma. Externally, it can be applied as a lotion to heal rashes, inflammation, sores and bruises.

Application and use: Infuse 1 handful of camomile flowers in 1 pint of boiling water for 10–15 minutes.

CARAWAY

Botanical name: *Carum carvi*.

Popular name: Caraway seed.

Habitat: Cultivated as culinary herb, and wild in grassy places.

Flora: Biennial, with white flowers June–July.

Folklore: The name derives from Arabic *karawiya*. It is known that this herb was cultivated by the ancient Egyptians, and its actual use by mankind may date back as far as 3000 BC. The cultivation of caraway seeds for medicinal purposes is mentioned in the Bible. In the seventeenth century caraway seeds were a popular confection, eaten dipped in sugar candy. In Shakespeare's day the roots of the plant were eaten as a vegetable, and Culpeper compared it favourably with parsnips, indicating that it was good for the digestion. Shakespeare in fact mentions the root in *The Merry Wives of Windsor* when a character says, 'In an arbour we will eat a last year's pippin of my own graffing with a dish of Caraway and so forth.' Caraway was often included in the wedding feast, or the seeds were thrown at the bride and groom as a good luck charm. As an aromatic plant it was also used to flavour liqueurs.

General medical properties: Antispasmodic, appetizer, carminative, stomachic and expectorant.

Specific properties: Caraway seeds contain an oil which has a beneficial effect on the gastric juices and prevents excessive flatulence; it is therefore recommended as a digestive and for treating lack of appetite. In addition the plant can be used to treat uterine cramps, and it promotes the flow of breast milk in nursing mothers. As a gargle it can be used to sooth the symptoms of laryngitis and sore throats in general.

Application and use: Infuse 3 teaspoons of crushed leaves in ½ cup of boiling water, or infuse 1 teaspoon of freshly crushed seeds in 1 cup of boiling water. Leave for 10–15 minutes. Cool, and drink a cup of the infusion 3 times a day.

CATNIP

Botanical name: *Nepeta cataria.*

Popular name: Catmint.

Habitat: Cultivated.

Flora: Perennial, with purple-white flowers June – September.

Folklore: Commonly called *Herba cateria* by the old folk healers, this plant has the uncanny power of attracting cats because of its distinctive smell. Whenever you see a patch of catnip in a country garden you will also see a cat sitting near it. So attracted by this herb are some cats that they will even eat the young shoots when they first appear in the early spring. Frequently catnip is used to stuff toy mice as playthings for cats. According to an old saying, the only sure way to grow catnip is to sow seeds; otherwise

> Set it, you won't get it.
> Sow it, they won't know it.

Today catnip is rarely used by herbalists for its medical properties, but it has always been highly regarded by practitioners of folk medicine.

General medical properties: Carminative, antispasmodic, sedative, astringent, stomachic and emmenagogue.

Specific properties: The use of this herb for medicinal purposes includes the treatment of infantile colic, anaemia, inhibited menstruation, diarrhoea, gastric upsets, insomnia, fevers, influenza, flatulence and nervousness. It contains an oil whose major ingredient is thymol, which has an antispasmodic effect useful for treating bronchitis. Externally, it can be applied to cuts, bruises and sores.

Application and use: Infuse 1 teaspoon of the herb in 1 cup of boiling water. Take 1–2 cups a day.

CAT'S FOOT

Botanical name: *Antennaria dioica.*

Popular names: Mountain everlasting, life everlasting, cud-weed, cotton weed.

Habitat: Woodland and meadows.

Flora: Perennial, with white and pink flowers May–August.

Folklore: The botanical name refers to its resemblance in shape to antennae. One of its popular names, cotton weed derives from the downy appearance of the leaves. The old herbalists used cat's foot as a remedy for mouth ulcers and to treat coughs.

General medical properties: Astringent, expectorant and mild diuretic.

Specific properties: Cat's foot can be used in cases of water retention and bronchitis, for treating mouth ulcers and as a gargle.

Application and use: Infuse 1 teaspoon of dried flowers in 1 cup of boiling water for 10–15 minutes. Take half a cup 3 times a day or as a gargle.

CAYENNE

Botanical name: *Capsicum annum.*

Popular names: Red pepper, chilli pepper.

Habitat: Cultivated.

Flora: Annual or biennial, with white flowers and distinctive red fruit.

Folklore: Cayenne peppers were introduced from North America in the fifteenth century, allegedly by the physician who sailed with Christopher Columbus to discover the New World. Because the plants are used to warm climates they have to be cultivated in greenhouses in the British Isles. The general name *Capsicum* derives from a Greek word meaning 'to bite', referring to its hot and pungent nature. The seventeenth- and eighteenth-century herbalists used cayenne pepper as a remedy for drunkenness.

General medical properties: Stimulant, tonic and digestive.

Specific properties: Tests with cayenne have indicated that it promotes the flow of gastric juices and saliva, and it is therefore both an appetizer and a digestive. It has also been recommended for treating nausea and as a cure for sore throats. Externally, it can be applied as a poultice to relieve sore or cramped muscles. It has the effect of mildly irritating the surface of the skin, which causes increased blood flow to the area and reduces inflammation. *Use with caution, since in concentrated form cayenne can cause irritation, especially on exposed skin.*

Application and use: ¾ teaspoon infused in 1 cup of boiling water.

CELERY

Botanical name: *Apium graveolens.*

Popular names: Common celery, wild celery.

Habitat: Cultivated and wild, in damp places near the sea.

Flora: Biennial, with white flowers July–November.

Folklore: Celery has been a popular vegetable since Roman times, even though in its wild form it tastes bitter. The cultivated celery eaten today was introduced by Italian gardeners in the Middle Ages. As well as being a popular salad plant, celery has also proved useful in folk remedies. It has been used as a cure for arthritis, rheumatism and gout, and was recommended for loss of appetite.

General medical properties: Antirheumatic, diuretic, carminative, sedative, appetizer and tonic.

Specific properties: In addition to its use in treating rheumatic pain, celery can also alleviate the state of depression which often accompanies this disease. It also acts as a urinary antiseptic, inhibits flatulence, promotes a good appetite and reduces obesity. Externally, it can be used to treat bruises.

Application and use: Infuse 1 teaspoon of seeds in ½ cup of boiling water, bring back to the boil and strain before use. Fresh celery juice extracted from the stems is also recommended. Take ½ cup 3 times daily.

CENTAURY

Botanical name: *Centaurium erythraea*.

Popular names: Feverwort, birthwort, common centaury.

Habitat: Woodland, fields and hedgerows.

Flora: Biennial or annual, with red flowers July–August.

Folklore: The name derives from the myth that Chiron the centaur used this herb to heal Hercules of an arrow wound. It was considered a sacred plant by the ancient Celtic druids, and preserved its magical aura into the Middle Ages. According to the medieval occultist Albertus Magnus, 'Magicians assured us that this herb has a singular virtue for if mixed with the blood of a female hoopoe and put in a lamp with oil all those present will see themselves upside down with their feet in the air.' Culpeper, with more inhibition than Albertus Magnus, assigned centaury to the astrological rulership of the sun, because 'their flowers open and shut as the Sun either showeth or hideth its face'. Today centaury is one of the herbal ingredients of vermouth.

General medical properties: Tonic, nervine, stomachic and appetizer.

Specific properties: Centaury is primarily used as a gastric stimulant, since its bitter ingredients have a stimulating effect on the stomach and gastro-intestinal system: it encourages appetite, and counteracts indigestion. It is also widely used as a tonic and for treating nervous conditions.

Application and use: Infuse 1 teaspoon of the dried herb in 1 cup of boiling water. Leave for 10 minutes. Take 1 cup before each meal.

CHERVIL

Botanical name: *Anthriscus cerefolium.*

Popular name: Garden chervil.

Habitat: Cultivated as a culinary herb.

Flora: Annual, with white flowers May–June.

Folklore: Chervil is a well-known culinary herb which was introduced from France, according to some botanists; however, others say it was brought to the British Isles by the Romans. It is used in sauces and soups, and as a garnish to fresh vegetables and salads. In the Middle Ages pregnant women were bathed in an infusion of this herb, which was believed to make them feel well. A lotion made from chervil juice was used by country-dwelling gentlewomen as a skin cleanser. Medically, it was used in folk remedies as a blood purifier.

General medical properties: Digestive, diuretic, depurative, tonic and expectorant.

Specific properties: Chervil juice can be used to treat skin disorders, gallstones, abscesses and sores, water retention, bronchitis and high blood pressure.

Application and use: Infuse 1 teaspoon of the fresh herb in ½ cup of boiling water. Take ½ cup a day. Alternatively, sprinkle the finely chopped herb over food.

CHICKWEED

Botanical name: *Stellaria media*.

Popular names: Starwort, adder's mouth, stitchwort, hen bite.

Habitat: Gardens, fields, hedgerows and wasteland.

Flora: Annual or biennial, with white flowers all year.

Folklore: As the list of possible habitats indicates, this is a prolific 'weed'. The botanical name, *Stellaria*, and the common name starwort, refer to the star-shaped flower. The name chickweed derives from the fact that traditionally this plant was used to feed chickens; it is also liked by rabbits, hamsters and gerbils. In the kitchen it can be prepared as a salad or cooked as a vegetable.

General medical properties: Vulnerary, antirheumatic, laxative, expectorant and emollient.

Specific properties: Chickweed is recommended for the treatment of skin diseases (especially where there is excessive itching), bronchitis, rheumatic pains, arthritis and period pains. Externally, the crushed stems and leaves can be used to heal open wounds, cuts, bruises and burns.

Application and use: Boil 1 teaspoon of the herb in 2 pints of water until only 1 pint remains. Take ½–1 cup a day. The crushed leaves can be made into a poultice or ointment for external application.

CHICORY

Botanical name: *Cichorium intybus.*

Popular name: Endive.

Habitat: Cultivated, and wild in grassy and waste places.

Flora: Perennial, with blue-violet flowers July–September

Folklore: Chicory is a well-known culinary herb which has recently received some popularity as a substitute for caffeine in coffee, especially in health food products. The common name endive comes from the Arabic *hendibeh*. The plant has a long history and is recorded in ancient Egypt, where its blanched leaves were used in salad, as they are often still used today. According to folk belief a sprig of chicory worn on the person had the magical power to unlock doors and to make the wearer invisible. The old herbalists used chicory principally as a tonic, and it was renowned by them for its stimulatory qualities.

General medical properties: Appetizer, tonic, digestive, laxative and diuretic.

Specific properties: The main use of the herb today is still as a tonic and mild stimulant, but it is also utilized to promote the appetite, especially after long illnesses, and to treat jaundice, gallstones, gastro-enteritis and sinus problems. Externally, it can be applied to cuts and bruises.

Application and use: Steep 1 teaspoon of the root or leaves in ½ cup of boiling water. Strain, and take 1–1½ cups of the resulting liquid a day. The boiled leaves or flowers can be applied externally as a poultice. *Use with caution, as prolonged dosage can affect the eyesight. If uncertain, consult a medical herbalist.*

CINQUEFOIL

Botanical name: *Potentilla anserina*.

Popular names: Wild tansy, silverweed, gooseweed, crampweed.

Habitat: Roadsides, marshy ground and pastures.

Flora: Perennial, with yellow flowers May–September.

Folklore: The early name of this plant was *Argentina*, meaning 'silver'; it belongs to a genus of plants with over three hundred different species, one of which, *Potentilla argentea*, retains the idea of the silver colour. The botanical name of the genus comes from Latin *potens*, 'powerful', a reference to the plant family's general astringent qualities; *anserina*, the specific name, means 'pertaining to geese' – it was thought that geese were attracted to the leaves as food. In the Middle Ages frogs were also recorded as being frequently found near cinquefoil, although no sensible reason has been offered to explain their liking for it. The name cinquefoil refers to its five distinct leaves; crampweed indicates that it was used in folk remedies to relieve the agony of muscular cramps. The medieval herbalists boiled the roots in milk as a cure-all, and the resulting juice was used to treat epilepsy. In magical lore this herb was said to have the power to ward off witches and evil spirits.

General medical properties: Astringent, antispasmodic, tonic and stomachic.

Specific properties: Cinquefoil can be used to treat piles, uterine and general muscular spasms, stomach pains and period discomfort, and as a gargle for mouth ulcers and sore throats. Externally, it can be used on cuts and wounds.

Application and use: Infuse 2 teaspoons of the root, or of the dried leaves or flowers, in 1 cup of boiling water. Take 1 cup 3 times daily.

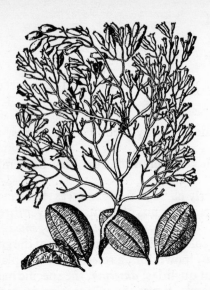

CLOVE

Botanical name: *Eugenia caryophyllata*.

Popular name: Clove.

Habitat: Imported from tropical countries.

Flora: Evergreen, with yellow flowers.

Folklore: Cloves were introduced into Europe as early as the sixth century as a culinary spice. Highly scented, they are still used as a flavouring in apple pies; in the sixteenth century they were included in body powders for their deodorant effect. Medically they have been used particularly in the relief of toothache because of their numbing nature.

General medical properties: Antiseptic and anaesthetic.

Specific properties: For the treatment of painful teeth.

Application and use: Apply oil of clove direct to the gum above or below the tooth.

COLTSFOOT

Botanical name: *Tussilago farfara.*

Popular names: Billsfoot, horsehoof, foalfoot, coughwort, bullsfoot, son-before-father.

Habitat: Wasteland and wet places.

Flora: Perennial, with yellowish flowers in early spring.

Folklore: Named after the shape of its leaves, coltsfoot has been recognized as a folk remedy for coughs since earliest times. The Greeks called it *bechion*, and the Romans knew it as *tussilago*, which can both be translated as 'cough plant'. When the Romans occupied Britain they sent back to Rome cough mixtures made of coltsfoot and flavoured with honey. Coltsfoot leaves are unusual because they appear after the flowers, which is why medieval herbalists nicknamed the herb *filius ante patrem* or 'the son before the father'. Coltsfoot was also a principal ingredient in herbal smoking mixtures, possibly because it had a soothing effect on the chest.

General medical properties: Emollient, demulcent, antispasmodic, diuretic and expectorant.

Specific properties: The primary use is for treating coughs, colds and bronchial disorders. It has a general calming action on inflamed respiratory tracts and can be used on asthmatic conditions. Externally, it can be applied in poultice form on sores and burns.

Application and use: Infuse 2 teaspoons of the dried flowers in 1 cup of boiling water. Drink warm 3 times a day. Freshly crushed leaves or flowers can be made into a poultice with honey and applied externally.

COLUMBINE

Botanical name: *Aquilegia vulgaris.*

Popular name: Common columbine.

Habitat: Woodland and scrub, and culivated as a garden flower.

Flora: Perennial, with blue and white flowers August–September.

Folklore: In the old herbals columbine was considered sacred to the planet Venus and the goddess of love; if you carried a posy of columbine, it was believed to elicit sincere affection from the person you loved. Culpeper said that a potion made from columbine seeds taken in wine made childbirth easier.

General medical properties: Astringent and diuretic.

Specific properties: Generally columbine is restricted to mouthwashes for sore gums and mouth ulcers, but it can also be used to ease childbirth and promotes urinary flow in cases of water retention.

Application and use: Steep 1 teaspoon in 1 cup of cold water. Bring to the boil and strain. Take 1 tablespoon 3 times a day.

COMFREY

Botanical name: *Symphytum officinale.*

Popular names: Knitbone, gumplant, healing herb, slippery root.

Habitat: Meadows and gardens.

Flora: Perennial, with whitish-purple flowers May–August.

Folklore: The common name of comfrey is derived from Latin *confirma* meaning 'joined together'. It was widely believed in ancient times that comfrey could help broken bones heal more quickly, hence its popular name of knitbone. The medical profession laughed at this claim until it was discovered that comfrey contains silica and albition, both substances which aid the fast healing of bone matter. Comfrey is an important animal feedstuff in many parts of the Third World and is also used as raw material for organic compost. Recent scientific tests have revealed that it is a natural source of vitamin B12 and is rich in protein – it is estimated that comfrey contains the same percentage of protein as soya beans and 10 per cent more than cheddar cheese. To date, attempts to extract this protein for human consumption have not proved successful.

General medical properties: Astringent, demulcent, vulnerary, expectorant and sedative.

Specific properties: Comfrey can be used as a cough remedy, for treating asthma, as a gargle for sore throats, and to treat tuberculosis and dysentery. Externally, a poultice of the leaves can be applied to cuts, wounds, bruises and varicose veins.

Application and use: Infuse 1 teaspoon of the rootstock in 1 cup of boiling water. Take 1 wineglass twice a day. A poultice made from the fresh leaves can be applied externally to sore breasts.

CORIANDER

Botanical name: *Coriandrum sativum.*

Popular name: Coriander.

Habitat: On bare ground, and cultivated.

Flora: Annual, with white and reddish flowers June–September.

Folklore: This plant, cultivated for over three thousand years, is mentioned in ancient Hindu scripts, in the medical texts of the Greek physicians, in the Bible, in the Ebers Papyrus of ancient Egypt and in almost every medieval herbal. Its name originated from Greek *koris*, 'bed bug', a reference to the similarly unpleasant smell of the unripe fruit. The fresh leaves are widely used for flavouring in various types of cookery, while the root can be cooked as a vegetable. The gastric juices are stimulated by chewing the seeds which are also used in making liqueurs, in curries and in baking.

General medical properties: Carminative, stimulant and appetizer.

Specific properties: Coriander is generally used to stimulate the appetite and cure flatulence. Applied externally, the bruised seeds offer relief from rheumatic pain.

Application and use: Infuse 1 teaspoon of the dried leaves or seeds in 1 cup of boiling water for 15 minutes. Take 1 cup daily.

CORNFLOWER

Botanical name: *Centaurea cyanus*.

Popular names: Bachelor's buttons, blue knapweed, blue burnet, bluebottle.

Habitat: Wild in cornfields and cultivated in gardens.

Flora: Annual, with blue flowers June–August.

Folklore: The cornflower gained its popular name of bachelor's buttons because it was often worn by young men in love; if the flower faded too quickly it was taken as an omen that the lady in question did not return that love. According to Greek myth the cornflower was originally a handsome boy who fell madly in love with the goddess Flora, whose festival was celebrated in the spring. The goddess changed the boy into a cornflower so that she would always have him by her side. Traditionally cornflowers are luck flowers. In folklore the cornflower was said to have the power to heal diseases of those with blue eyes. Although it was once a common sight in English cornfields, the herbicides of modern agriculture are fast making it a rarity in its natural environment.

General medical properties: Diuretic, tonic and astringent.

Specific properties: Cornflowers are recommended for treating eye irritations, conjunctivitis and weak eyesight. They can also be used in cases of water retention and as a general tonic.

Application and use: Infuse 1 oz of dried flowers in 2 pints of boiling water. Strain, cool, and take 1 cup before meals.

COUCH GRASS

Botanical name: *Elymus repens.*

Popular names: Twitchgrass, witch grass.

Habitat: Wasteland.

Flora: Perennial, with purple flowers June–October.

Folklore: Although hated by gardeners because it is very difficult to eradicate, couch grass has a long history as a medicinal plant dating back to ancient Greece and Rome. Sick dogs are known to seek out the plant and eat it to cause vomiting. In the past the roasted root has been used as a substitute for coffee and as a replacement for bread during periods of famine. The medieval herbalists used couch grass to treat inflamed bladders, painful urination and water retention; recent scientific tests have indicated that it does possess a strong diuretic action. Other tests have proved that it has antibiotic qualities, too.

General medical properties: Antiseptic, antibacterial and diuretic.

Specific properties: Recommended for the treatment of water retention, in cystitis and as a urinary antiseptic.

Application and use: Infuse 1 teaspoon of the root in 1 cup of boiling water. Cool and strain. Take 1 cup a day.

COWSLIP

Botanical name: *Primula veris*.

Popular names: Palsy wort, St Peter's herb, herb Peter.

Habitat: Meadows and marshy land.

Flora: Perennial, with yellow flowers May–June.

Folklore: Cowslips derive their common name from the Old English *cusloppe* or cowslop, because they grew in fields where domesticated animals were grazed. Its generic name comes from Latin *primus*, first, referring to the fact that it flowers in the early spring. The popular name of herb Peter or St Peter's herb originated in the myth that the flower sprang up on the ground where the saint dropped the keys to Heaven. The medieval herbalists regarded the cowslip as a safe sedative for those suffering from insomnia. It was also said to cure the palsy, a form of paralysis with involuntary tremors – hence another of its names. Although once widely used in folk remedies, by the 1870s its popularity had declined. In the nineteenth century cowslips were used to garland maypoles and were scattered on the village green for country dances. Cowslip was also a major ingredient in country wines, fermented with sugar, honey and lemon juice. The roots were also used in the brewing of orthodox wines and beers to improve the flavour of the finished product. The candied flowers were used for cake decorations and were popular as confectionery. In folklore the cowslip was regarded as the home of elves and fairies, hence Puck's lines in Shakespeare's *A Midsummer Night's Dream*:

> Where the bee sucks there suck I,
> In a Cowslip's bell I lie: There I couch when owls do cry

General medical properties: Sedative, nervine, anti-spasmodic, expectorant and narcotic.

Specific properties: Cowslip is used to cure insomnia, ease bronchial coughs and act as a general nerve sedative.

Application and use: *Use with caution, as cowslips have irritant qualities to which allergy sufferers may prove sensitive.* Infuse ½ oz of leaves or flowers in 1 pint of water. Drink 1–2 cups a day.

DAISY

Botanical name: *Bellis perennis.*

Popular name: Eye-of-the-day.

Habitat: Wild in pastures, and cultivated.

Flora: Perennial, with yellow and white flowers March–October.

Folklore: The humble daisy is held in high regard by horticulturists because it manufactures lime and so enriches the soil. Chaucer called it the eye-of-the-day because it opens its flower when the sun shines and closes it at sunset. The childhood custom of making daisy chains is of great antiquity: it may date from sacrificial offerings of flowers made to the old pagan gods.

General medical properties: Expectorant, astringent and diuretic.

Specific properties: Daisies are recommended to help alleviate kidney disorders, rheumatism, arthritis, bronchitis and diarrhoea.

Application and use: Infuse 1 teaspoon of the dried herb for 10 minutes in a cup of boiling water. Drink 1 cup 2–3 times a day.

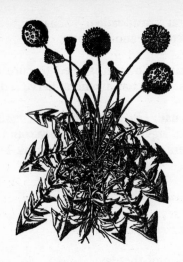

DANDELION

Botanical name: *Taraxacum officinale*.

Popular names: Lion's tooth, priest's crown, puffball.

Habitat: Wasteland.

Flora: Perennial, with yellow flowers in early summer followed by distinctive puffball of seeds.

Folklore: The common name of dandelion is derived from the French dent de lion or lion's teeth, which the leaves were said to resemble. The Tudors gave it the rather cruder nickname of piss-in-the-bed, a reference to its ability to increase the flow of urine. Children have always blown the seeds from its puffball to tell the time; however, it is said that if all the seeds are blown away the unfortunate child will be rejected by its mother. In country lore, to see the seeds blown free of the puffball by the wind is claimed to be a sign of rain coming. The plant was also used in a popular rustic love charm: a single girl plucked a fresh dandelion and blew the fluffy head; the number of blows it took to disperse all the seeds indicated the number of years she would have to wait before getting married. To dream of a dandelion is a portent of difficult times ahead. Ideally, dandelions should be gathered on Midsummer's Eve (23 June) when they were supposed to have the power to ward off the evil spirits believed to be abroad on that night.

Apart from being a medical plant the dandelion has also been used for food. Its blanched leaves are used in salads, and the roots provide a coffee substitute as sold in health food shops. There is very little mention of the herb in the classical world, but it is known that the Arabs used it in the eleventh century. A Russian variety of the plant was grown during the Second World War because its roots exuded a latex material from which rubber was made; the British plant provides only small quantities of this product, insufficient for commercial use. In scientific tests dandelion roots have been proved to increase bile secretion, which might prove useful in the treatment of hepatitis.

General medical properties: Diuretic, laxative, tonic, anti-rheumatic, expectorant and appetizer.

Specific properties: The dandelion is mainly recommended for use as a diuretic to cure water retention. It can also be used in the treatment of chest congestion, jaundice, rheumatic pain, gout, constipation, diabetes, circulatory disorders, insomnia, anaemia and as an anticholesterol agent.

Application and use: Steep 2 teaspoons of the herb in 1 cup of cold water. Boil, cool and strain. Take ½ cup a day, lukewarm or cold.

DILL

Botanical name: Anethum graveolens.

Popular names: Dilly, dillweed, common dill, garden dill.

Habitat: On wasteland, and cultivated as a culinary herb.

Flora: Annual, with yellow flowers in June.

Folklore: The common name of dill originates in a word in the Indo-European group of languages meaning 'to blossom', and is said to have originated in Asia. It has been used as a medical plant for centuries and is mentioned in the Bible. In folklore dill has traditionally been regarded as an antidote to witchcraft: according to the old country rhyme, 'Vervain and Dill hinderith witches of their will.' It was also regarded as a plant with aphrodisiac properties, and was a favoured ingredient in medieval love potions. Dill water is still included in recipes for gripe water to be administered to children. In the kitchen dill can be a flavouring or garnish in soup and sauces, with fish and in cakes and pastries. It is also used as a perfume in cosmetic soaps.

General medical properties: Carminative, appetizer, antispasmodic, nervine, stomachic, stimulant and galactagogue.

Specific properties: Dill is said to cure flatulence, insomnia, colic and indigestion, and to increase the appetite. It also promotes breast milk in nursing mothers. The seeds, chewed, are recommended for halitosis.

Application and use: Steep 2 teaspoons of the seeds in 1 cup of boiling water for 10–15 minutes. Take ½ cup 2–4 times per day.

DOCK

Botanical name: *Rumex obtusifolius*.

Popular names: Broad-leaved dock, herb Patience.

Habitat: Wasteland.

Flora: Perennial, with greenish flowers June–September.

Folklore: Dock leaves are an old country cure for nettle stings, and the plant is often found in the vicinity of a nettle bed. The general use of the dock family in folk remedies is as a laxative and for jaundice.

General medical properties: Astringent, tonic, purgative and cathartic.

Specific properties: This plant can be used as an all-purpose purging agent, especially in cases of liver disorder. Externally, it can be used to treat skin diseases such as ringworm and scabies. In small doses it is regarded as a tonic.

Application and use: *Only on the advice of a medical herbalist, as contact for long periods can create skin allergy and overdosing causes nausea.*

DOG ROSE

Botanical name: *Rosa canina*.

Popular names: Briar rose, queen of flowers.

Habitat: Woodland and hedgerows.

Flora: Perennial shrub, with white or pale pink flowers June–August.

Folklore: This flowering shrub gained its popular name of dog rose because medieval herbalists of the seventeenth and eighteenth centuries used it to treat the bites of rabid dogs. Pliny the Elder said that the ancient name for Britain – Albion – was derived from Latin *alba*, meaning 'white', because the island was covered with wild white roses. Rosehips, a natural source of vitamin C, were used in folk remedies to treat colds and influenza; rosehip syrup was manufactured in large quantities during the Second World War when other sources of vitamin C, such as oranges, were unavailable.

General medical properties: Laxative, diuretic, astringent and tonic.

Specific properties: Rosehip syrup is recommended for the prevention and treatment of colds, influenza and bronchitis. It can also be used as a general tonic, for constipation and infections of the gall bladder.

Application and use: Infuse 2½ teaspoons of rosehips in a cup of boiling water. Simmer for ten minutes. Strain and take 1 cup daily.

ELDER

Botanical name: *Sambucus nigra.*

Popular name: Black elder.

Habitat: Woods and gardens.

Flora: Perennial shrub or tree, with yellow-white flowers July–September.

Folklore: The elder was known to the ancient Egyptians and has a long history in folk medicine. Elderflower water is still used in modern cosmetic preparations, and is recommended as a skin cleanser and a treatment for sunburn. Medieval herbalists and folk healers used elderberries to bring on menstruation. Until comparatively recently elderflower and peppermint were widely used in a rural folk remedy for coughs and colds. Elderflowers and elderberries both produce a very light, enjoyable wine popular among country people. The fruit can also be used in conserves, jams and pies.

For various reasons the elder was regarded with awe by country folk, who thought it was an unlucky tree to have in the garden despite its many advantages. If a tree was cut down it was believed that the Elder Mother who lived inside it would wreak havoc in the lives of those responsible. This folk belief dates back to the pagan worship of the Moon Goddess, who had the elder as her sacred tree. If you gathered elder branches on May Day, it was believed that pieces of it could be used to cure the bite of a rabid dog. However, the tree could only be cut safely by repeating the following charm before touching it with your saw: 'Old girl give me of thy wood and I will give you some of mine when I grow into a tree.' This simple trick was said to save the cutter from a dire fate for daring to interfere with the Elder Mother.

General medical properties: Diuretic, purgative, antispasmodic and laxative.

Specific properties: Elder's berries, flowers, leaves and bark can be used to treat constipation, arthritis, influenza, hay fever, sinus trouble, fevers and catarrh. Externally, they are helpful for bruises, chilblains and sprains.

Application and use: Infuse 2 tablespoon of flowers in 1 cup of boiling water. Take 3 cups a day, hot. Infuse fresh berries in boiling water for 2–3 minutes and extract the juice. Take 1 wineglass, diluted with water, a day. *Use with caution*.

ELECAMPANE

Botanical name: *Inula helenium*.

Popular name: Elfwort, scabwort.

Habitat: Damp places, woodland and hedgerows.

Flora: Perennial, with yellow flowers June–September.

Folklore: The specific name, *helenium,* derives from Helen who was carried off to Troy by Paris in classical mythology; where her tears fell on the ground this flower is said to have sprung up. A sacred plant to the ancient Celts, it was known to the Anglo-Saxons and used by the medieval Welsh herbalists. Its other popular names of elfwort and scabwort may indicate respectively a connection with the fairies and its use in curing skin diseases. Gerard recommended its use for 'the shortness of breath' and dealing with persistent coughs; he claimed that the plant purged the chest of phlegm and mucus. In medieval times the flowers were candied and eaten as a confection, and elecampane is still used in the flavouring of some European wines and liqueurs.

General medical properties: Expectorant, tonic and antibiotic.

Specific properties: The chief use of elecampane is as an expectorant for dealing with bronchial coughs. It is also used in cases of water retention and as an antiseptic. In addition it promotes menstruation and is a tonic and appetizer, although these are only minor uses.

Application and use: Infuse 1 teaspoon of the root in 1½ pints of boiling water for 15 minutes. Drink 1–2 cups a day as required.

EYEBRIGHT

Botanical name: *Euphrasia officinalis.*

Popular name: Meadow eyebright.

Habitat: Meadows and pastures.

Flora: Annual, with white flowers June–September.

Folklore: The generic name originates in a Greek word meaning 'gladness'. It seems to have been unknown to European herbalists until it was introduced in a herbal dated 1305, although it was known in the classical world. Culpeper assigned this herb to the zodiac sign of Leo (21 July–21 August) and said that it strengthened the brain. Gerard recommended it for 'feeble eyes' and, as its common name suggests, this was its principal use in folk medicine. In ancient Iceland the plant's juice was used to treat serious eye disorders; in medieval Scotland folk healers mixed its juice with milk and applied it as a lotion to the eyes, using a feather. Folk herbalists also used eyebright to restore a bad memory and in cases of vertigo.

General medical properties: Astringent, anti-catarrhal and anti-inflammatory.

Specific properties: Eyebright can be used to cure eye problems, sinus disorders, catarrh, allergies and inflammation.

Application and use: Infuse 1 teaspoon of the dried herb in 1 cup of boiling water for 10 minutes. Cool, strain and take 1 cup 3 times a day or use as an eyebath.

FAT HEN

Botanical name: *Chenopodium album.*

Popular names: White goosefeet, pigweed.

Habitat: Wasteland.

Flora: Annual, with greenish-white flowers June–September.

Folklore: The generic name derives from Greek *khenopodion*, meaning 'goosefoot', a reference to the shape of its leaves. Fat hen is related to spinach and is an edible vegetable which was included in the human diet from Stone Age times to the nineteenth century. The seeds can be crushed to make flour, and the leaves can be cooked like spinach or eaten raw in salads. The plant has also been widely used as animal feed.

General medical properties: Purgative.

Specific properties: Fat hen plant is rich in iron, calcium and vitamins B1 and C. It can therefore be used in cases of anaemia and vitamin C deficiency, and as a laxative to cure constipation.

Application and use: Infuse 1 teaspoon of the dried herb in 1 cup of boiling water. Take 1 cup a day.

FENNEL

Botanical name: *Foeniculum vulgare.*

Popular names: Common fennel, sweet fennel.

Habitat: Wild on wasteland, and cultivated as a culinary herb.

Flora: Perennial or biennial (occasionally annual), with yellow flowers July–October.

Folklore: The plant's generic name comes from Latin *foeniculum*, which means 'little hay' and refers to the appearance of the dried leaves. Fennel was introduced into northern and western Europe by the occupying Roman armies. The ancient Egyptians, Greeks, Chinese and Hindus used it for both its culinary qualities and medicinal properties. Pliny the Elder cites over twenty herbal remedies containing fennel, and the Greek physicians said that it increased milk flow in nursing mothers. It is one of the nine sacred herbs mentioned in the famous Anglo-Saxon charm. According to a country saying, fennel should never be cultivated but only gathered from the wild: 'Sow Fennel, sow trouble' was the rustic advice. Despite this, fennel has been a popular feature of kitchen herb gardens for centuries. It is used in soups and sauces, and as a garnish for fish. The roots and stems may be eaten as a vegetable, and the seeds are used in liqueur manufacture. In folk belief, a few fennel seeds placed in the keyhole of a haunted house kept ghosts away. In magical lore fennel was believed to be able to restore libido to the impotent and frigid, and for this reason it was often included in medieval love charms and potions.

General medical properties: Antispasmodic, carminative, diuretic, stomachic, stimulant, expectorant and galactagogue.

Specific properties: Fennel has a strong smell of aniseed. It can be recommended for colic, flatulence, indigestion, bronchitis, obesity, jaundice, sore throats, bed-wetting, gall bladder disorders, colic, earache and toothache. It also has uses in veterinary medicine. The seeds, boiled in barley water, are said to increase the flow of breast milk.

Application and use: *Use with caution, as overdosing can affect the nervous system and the fresh leaves are an irritant.* Infuse 2 teaspoons of the crushed leaves or seeds in 1 cup of boiling water for 10 minutes. Take 3 times a day.

FENUGREEK

Botanical name: *Trigonella foenum-graecum.*

Popular name: Greek hay.

Habitat: Wasteland, and cultivated.

Flora: Annual, with pink flowers June–July.

Folklore: Originally fenugreek was extensively cultivated in the ancient world as an animal feedstuff, hence its common and specific names, Greek hay and *foenum-graecum*. It is believed that the herb was introduced into medieval Europe by the Benedictine order of monks, but it was not mentioned in any English herbal until the sixteenth century. Fenugreek was used by the famous Arab physicians, but the Egyptians and Hindus cultivated it for food. In the Middle Ages it is recorded that fenugreek was added to inferior hay because of its pleasant smell. Culpeper assigned rulership of the herb to the planet Mercury, which rules Gemini (21 May–20 June) and Virgo (22 August–22 September). He claimed that the bruised leaves, placed on top of the head, cured vertigo. Seventeenth-century apothecaries recommended that after giving birth women should sit over the fumes from a decoction of this herb, with their legs open, to help expel the placenta. Today fenugreek is widely used in veterinary medicine, in chutney and curries, and as a substitute for coffee.

General medical properties: Emollient, vulnerary, tonic, expectorant and demulcent.

Specific properties: Fenugreek has always been renowned for expelling poisons and unwanted waste materials from the human body. It can also be used as a cure for bronchitis, a gargle for sore throats and a general tonic. Externally, it is recommended for treating wounds, sores and boils.

Application and use: Infuse 1 teaspoon of the seeds in 1 cup of boiling water for 10 minutes. Use one cup 3 times daily.

FEVERFEW

Botanical name: *Tanacetum parthenium*.

Popular names: Flirtwort, feverwort, featherfoil.

Habitat: Farmland.

Flora: Perennial, with yellow flowers June–July.

Folklore: The common name of feverfew is derived from Latin *febrifugia*, which means a plant which has the ability to drive out fevers. According to the old herbalists and folk healers, feverfew was used to bring on menstruation and for expelling the placenta after childbirth; it was also used in cases of stillbirth. Culpeper stated that this herb was ruled by the goddess Venus and had been provided by her to aid womankind. When its leaves are crushed it gives off an unpleasant smell which repels insects.

General medical properties: Tonic, sedative, mild laxative and emmenagogue.

Specific properties: Recent research has indicated that feverfew is very efficacious in the treatment of headaches and migraine. It can also be used in cases of colic, flatulence, indigestion, colds, influenza, alcoholic poisoning and inhibited menstrual flow.

Application and use: Infuse 1 teaspoon of the dried leaves or flowers in 1 cup of boiling water, and take 1 cup daily.

FIGWORT

Botanical name: *Scrophularia nodosa.*

Popular name: Pilewort, throat-wort, heal all.

Habitat: Wet places, ditches and woodland.

Flora: Perennial, with greenish-brown flowers June–July.

Folklore: It is believed that the name figwort is a corruption of Latin *ficus*, 'fig'. In the classical world it was used as a herbal cure for piles, which resemble figs! Culpeper states that figwort is ruled by the planet Venus and the zodiac sign of Taurus (21 April–20 May). He recommended its use to cure the skin disease known as the King's Evil in his day but now known as scrofula. Folk healers believed that the beneficial action of this plant on the liver would cure any skin disorder.

General medical properties: Diuretic, mild laxative, cardiac stimulant.

Specific properties: Figwort can be used to cure sore throats, ease constipation and stimulate the heart, and to alleviate water retention. Externally, it can be used to treat all skin diseases and helps reduce the swellings of bruises.

Application and use: Infuse 1 teaspoon of the dried root stock or flowers in 1 cup of boiling water. Take 1–2 cups a day.

FLAG
See Purple Flag, Sweet Flag.

FLAX

Botanical name: *Linum usitatissimum.*

Popular name: Linseed.

Habitat: Grassland, and cultivated.

Flora: Annual, with blue flowers June–July.

Folklore: It is estimated that flax has been cultivated for use in making linen for at least three thousand years. The ancient Egyptians used flax-derived linen to wrap their mummies, and it was imported into northern and western Europe by the Romans. The first recorded use of flax in western Europe was in Ireland *c*. AD 500. To ensure a good crop of flax, farmers used to ring the local church bells on Ascension Day. Flax oil has many uses in modern industry, including the manufacture of paints and varnish.

General medical properties: Demulcent, emollient and laxative.

Specific properties: Medically, the linseed oil derived from the flax seeds has emollient properties, both internally and externally, and is effective on burns. The plant is used to treat bronchitis and lung disorders, and for easing childbirth and constipation.

Application and use: Infuse 1 teaspoon of ripe seeds in 2 pints of water. Boil until only 1 pint remains. Sip occasionally during the day. For external use mix crushed seeds with hot water and apply as a poultice.

FUMITORY

Botanical name: *Fumaria officinalis*.

Popular name: Earth smoke.

Habitat: Wasteland, fields and gardens.

Flora: Annual, with reddish-purple flowers May–September.

Folklore: Expert opinion differs considerably on the origin of this plant's name. According to some, the classical writers thought that it grew from 'the vapours of the Earth'. Other sources say that its grey leaves look like wisps of smoke rising from the ground. Alternatively, it was claimed that the smoke derived from burning its leaves had magical powers and could drive away evil spirits. Folk healers believed that its use to improve the eyesight had the side-effect of causing the eyes to water, as if they had been exposed to smoke. In the Middle Ages young women washed themselves with a decoction of fumitory to make skin blemishes vanish.

General medical properties: Diuretic, laxative, alterative and stomachic.

Specific properties: Used for serious skin diseases, cleansing the kidneys and to treat conjunctivitis.

Application and use: *Toxic. Use only under the direction of a medical herbalist.*

GARLIC

Botanical name: *Allium ursinum.*

Popular name: Wild garlic, ramsons.

Habitat: Wild in hedgerows and woodland, and cultivated.

Flora: Perennial, with white flowers in summer.

Folklore: The common name originates in the Anglo-Saxon *gar*, meaning 'lance', and *leac*, meaning 'pot herb'. In common folklore garlic bulbs hung around the neck traditionally ward off vampires. Country people often grew a patch of garlic in their gardens as a protection against the spells of black witches. Garlic has always been recognized as one of the most important natural folk remedies. The ancient Egyptians valued garlic bulbs so highly that they ordered a daily ration of them to be fed to the builders of the pyramids to give them strength. In ancient China the plant was used by physicians as a cure for leprosy. During the plague outbreaks in the Middle Ages, garlic was widely used as an antiseptic. This use persisted as late as the First World War, when troops in the trenches were treated with garlic to prevent their wounds from becoming septic. The garlic plant belongs to the same botanical genus as the onion, and is widely used in cooking, especially in European countries.

General medical properties: Expectorant, diuretic, nervine and antibacterial.

Specific properties: Scientists at New York State University have recently discovered that garlic contains a chemical substance called ajeone, which acts as a blood thinner; they believe that it can be used to treat circulatory complaints such as arteriosclerosis and blood clots which cause strokes. Garlic is also recommended for treating colds, sinus disorders, bronchitis, asthma and colic. It lowers blood pressure, purifies the blood and acts as a nerve sedative. Externally, it can be used to treat chilblains.

Application and use: For general use, take ½ teaspoon of garlic juice pressed from fresh bulbs 2–3 times a day. For coughs, eat grated bulbs mixed with honey. To treat asthma, boil a large quantity of bulbs in water until they are soft, then add as much vinegar as there is water left over. Add some sugar, and boil again until a syrup is formed. Take 2–3 teaspoons a day, as required.

GENTIAN
See Great Yellow Gentian.

GOLDEN ROD

Botanical name: *Solidago virgaurea*.

Popular names: Aaron's rod, woundwort.

Habitat: Wild in woodland and heathland, and cultivated in gardens.

Flora: Perennial, with yellow flowers July–October.

Folklore: Golden ród was cultivated by the Arabs, who recognized its important medical uses. Its popular name of Aaron's rod suggests that it may have been known to the Hebrews for similar reasons. In the fifteenth and sixteenth centuries herbalists used golden rod to heal wounds, hence another popular name.

General medical properties: Astringent, diuretic, anti-catarrhal, antispasmodic and antiseptic.

Specific properties: Golden rod is used for treating catarrh, dissolving kidney stones, cleansing wounds and curing water retention.

Application and use: Infuse 2 teaspoons of the dried flowers in 1 cup of boiling water for 15 minutes. Take 3 times a day.

GOOSE GRASS

Botanical name: *Galium aparine.*

Popular name: Cleavers.

Habitat: Fields and hedgerows.

Flora: Annual, with white or whitish-green flowers in summer.

Folklore: The popular name refers to the clinging action of the stems, which are covered in tiny prickles. In folk medicine the herb was used to treat skin diseases. The dried plant can be used to make a herbal tea, and is also recommended as a coffee substitute.

General medical properties: Vulnerary and diuretic.

Specific properties: This plant is recommended for lowering blood pressure and reducing the temperature in fevers. It is also used for treating water retention and cystitis. Externally, it can be used to heal wounds and skin diseases.

Application and use: Infuse 1 teaspoon of the dried flowers in 1 cup of boiling water for 15 minutes. Take 1 cup a day.

GREATER CELANDINE

Botanical name: *Chelidonium majus.*

Popular names: Jewel weed, snap weed, touch-me-not, felon-wort, swallow wort.

Habitat: Wasteland and hedgerows.

Flora: Although a member of the poppy family, with which it shares narcotic properties, this wild flower is sometimes confused with the buttercup, probably because lesser celandine (*Ranunculus ficaria*), to which greater celandine is not related, somewhat resembles the buttercup in appearance. Greater celandine's botanical name comes from the Greek *khelidon*, meaning 'swallow', a reference to the popular belief that the herb flowers when the swallows arrive from North Africa in the summer. Pliny the Elder, the Roman writer on herbalism who was renowned for his speculative stories, claimed that it was so named because 'swallows cured their young ones' eyes that were hurt by bringing this herb and putting it on them'. As greater celandine is frequently found growing on waste ground near human habitation, some authorities have taken this as a sign that it was cultivated for medical purposes. In magical lore during the Middle Ages it was believed that anyone who carried a bunch of greater celandine flowers and the heart of a mole could conquer his enemies and win law suits with ease. On a more mundane level, it was utilized by gypsies as a foot refresher.

General medical properties: Narcotic, purgative and stomachic.

Specific properties: The use of this herb is restricted to its purgative qualities and for treating skin diseases. *As it is very toxic it should be used with extreme caution.*

Application and use: *Strictly only on the advice, and under the direction, of a qualified medical herbalist.*

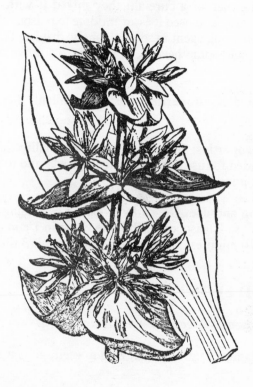

GREAT YELLOW GENTIAN

Botanical name: *Gentiana lutea.*

Popular names: Felwort, bitter root, bald Mary.

Habitat: Hilly pastures and woodland.

Flora: Perennial, with yellow flowers in August.

Folklore: This plant, legendary in folk medicine, was named after the ancient King Gentius, who lived in what is now Yugoslavia in the first century BC; he was allegedly the first person to discover its medical uses. It was widely used for medical purposes by both the Greeks and Arabs, probably on account of its renowned bitterness. Medieval herbalists regarded Gentian as a cure-all; they mixed it with honey to disguise its taste and used it as an antidote to poison. Today it is used as a bittering agent in some alcoholic drinks. The plant is long-lived, and some have been known to survive for nearly fifty years.

General medical properties: Gastric stimulant, digestive and appetizer.

Specific properties: Because of its bitter quality this herb is recommended for use as an appetite improver and to stimulate the gastric juices.

Application and use: *Use with caution, as overdosing can cause nausea.* Infuse 1 teaspoon of the dried root in 1 cup of boiling water for 10 minutes. Drink 1 cup before meals 3 times a day.

GROUND ELDER

Botanical name: *Aegopodium podagraria.*

Popular names: Herb Gerard, bishopweed, gout weed, goatweed.

Habatit: Hedgerows and roadsides.

Flora: Perennial, with white flowers in summer.

Folklore: The botanical name is derived from Greek *aigos*, 'goat, and *podos*, 'foot', and Latin *podagra*, 'gout'. In the Middle Ages folk healers recommended this persistent weed, which is the bane of gardeners, as a herbal remedy for gout. Its young leaves can be cooked as a vegetable or eaten raw in salads.

General medical properties: Diuretic, sedative and pain reliever.

Specific properties: It is mainly used for treating gout and sciatic pain and also rheumatism, also in cases of water retention to promote urine.

Application and use: As a diuretic, infuse 1 teaspoon of the fresh leaves in 1 cup of boiling water for 15 minutes. Take 1 cup a day. For external use, apply fresh leaves as a poultice to painful areas.

GROUND IVY

Botanical name: *Glechoma hederacea.*

Popular names: Cat's foot, alehoof, Jack-in-the-hedge, Gill-creep-by-the-ground.

Habitat: Hedgerows.

Flora: Perennial, with blue-purple flowers in late spring and early summer.

Folklore: Despite its common name, this plant is not a member of the ivy family. It was used in Saxon times as an additive in beer, and was recommended by medieval practitioners of folk medicine for the cure of urinary infections and persistent coughs.

General medical properties: Astringent, expectorant, anti-catarrhal and diuretic.

Specific properties: Used for treating catarrh, bronchitis and cystitis, for easing sciatic pain and as a gargle for sore throats.

Application and use: Infuse 1 teaspoon of the dried leaves in 1 cup of boiling water for 15 minutes. Take 3 times a day.

GROUNDSEL

Botanical name: *Senecio vulgaris.*

Popular names: Birdseed, ragwort.

Habitat: Fields and gardens.

Flora: Annual, with yellow flowers in summer.

Folklore: This plant is disliked by gardeners because it spreads quickly and is difficult to eradicate from cultivated land; its common name comes from an Old English word translated as 'ground swallower'. Pliny the Elder recommended groundsel for the treatment of toothache: he suggested that the afflicted person rubbed the tooth with the plant and then replaced it in the ground; if the plant rerooted itself, the tooth would cease to hurt. In folk medicine this plant was widely used to treat female disorders, especially painful periods; the medieval herbalists used it to help young girls who were going through the trauma of their first period at the onset of puberty. It was once used as birdseed, hence another of its popular names.

General medical properties: Stomachic, purgative, laxative and astringent.

Specific properties: In addition to the relief of period pains groundsel also acts as a laxative and for stomach ache. Externally, it can be used as an antiseptic lotion for cleansing wounds and to treat bleeding gums.

Application and use: *Large doses can cause liver problems. Use only as directed by a medical herbalist.*

GYPSYWORT

Botanical name: *Lycopus europaeus.*

Popular Name: Gypsyweed.

Habitat: Marshes and ditches.

Flora: Perennial, with white and purple flowers in July–September.

Folklore: Gypsywort is so named because the Romany tribes extracted from the plant a black dye which has been used for centuries to colour linen.

General medical properties: Cardiac, sedative and anti-haemorrhagic.

Specific properties: In folk medicine this herb has been used to prevent blood clotting, as a sedative in heart conditions and high blood pressure, and for reducing the pulse rate in over-active thyroid conditions.

Application and use: Infuse 1 teaspoon of the dried flowers in 1 cup of boiling water for 10 minutes. Take one cup three times a day.

HAWTHORN

Botanical name: *Crataegus monogyna*.

Popular names: May, whitethorn.

Habitat: Woodland and hedgerows.

Flora: Perennial tree, with white flowers in May.

Folklore: The hawthorn was once highly regarded as a magical tree sacred to the fairies and the pagan fertility goddesses of pre-Christian times. The Church also looked on the tree with respect, as it was supposed to have been the origin of the crown of thorns worn by Jesus on the cross. It was said to be unlucky to bring hawthorn blossom into a house before May Day. Laid above the lintels of doors, hawthorn branches warded off witches, evil spirits and lightning. As Sir John Mandeville said in 1350, 'The white thorn hath many virtues for he that bearest it on him none manner of tempest shall harm him. [If it] be in the house where you are in then none evil ghost shall enter.' The virtue of the hawthorn to protect from thunderstorms is recorded in this old saying:

> Beware of the oak
> It draws the stroke.
> Around the ash
> It courts the flash.
> Creep under the thorn
> It will save you from harm.

In the Middle Ages peasant girls bathed in hawthorn dew on May Morning to improve their complexions. The strange smell of the hawthorn blossom made some country people say that it carried the Great Plague, while others claim that the odour has aphrodisiac qualities.

General medical properties: Tonic, nervine and cardiac stimulant.

Specific properties: Hawthorn berries are used in folk medicine as a general tonic and heart stimulant. The tree is also recommended for the treatment of hypertension, sore throats and chilblains.

Application and use: Infuse 2 teaspoons of berries in 1 cup of boiling water for 15 minutes. Take 3 times a day.

HEATHER

Botanical name: *Calluna vulgaris*.

Popular name: Ling.

Habitat: Heaths and moorland.

Flora: Evergreen shrub, with pink flowers August–October.
Folklore: The generic name comes from a Greek word meaning 'to sweep': in the old days besom heads were often made from

the stiff branches. In folk belief heather has always been regarded as a lucky plant to grow in the garden; its use as a good luck charm by the gypsies is well known, and continues to this day.

General medical properties: Astringent, antiseptic, sedative and diuretic.

Specific properties: It is used as a sedative in cases of insomnia, as an antiseptic for cleansing wounds, and for urinary infections. Externally, it can be used to treat skin diseases.

Application and use: Infuse 1 teaspoon of the dried flowers in 1 cup of boiling water for 15 minutes. Take 1 cup a day.

HEDGE MUSTARD

Botanical name: *Sisymbrium officinale*.

Popular names: Wiry Jack, singer's plant.

Habitat: Fields, wasteland and hedgerows.

Flora: Perennial, with yellow flowers April–November.

Folklore: The Greeks used this plant for medical purposes, believing that an infusion of it mixed with honey was an antidote for all known poisons. In folk medicine hedge mustard was recommended for its ability to soothe sore throats, and was therefore used by public speakers and professional singers. It was once used in sauces, but its strong flavour makes it an acquired taste.

General medical properties: Diuretic, expectorant, tonic, stomachic and laxative.

Specific properties: The juice and flowers are recommended for use in bronchitis, water retention, constipation and stomach upsets, and as a general tonic and revitalizer.

Application and use: *Use with caution. Overdosing can affect the heart. It must not be used to treat old people or children.* Steep 1 teaspoon of the dried flowers in ½ cup of boiling water for 5 minutes. Take 1–2 cups a day.

HERB ROBERT

Botanical name: *Geranium robertianum.*

Popular names: Red robin, St Robert's herb.

Habitat: Woodland and wasteland.

Flora: Annual or biennial, with pink or red flowers June–September.

Folklore: In the Middle Ages this plant was regarded as sacred to St Robert. It was also believed to be the special herb of the fairies, and was associated with hobgoblins. Herb Robert was widely used in medieval folk medicine.

General medical properties: Astringent, diuretic and sedative.

Specific properties: Used to treat sensitive skin complaints, as a lotion for eye trouble, for stopping diarrhoea, as a gargle for mouth ulcers and sore throats, and externally to reduce swellings and bruises.

Application and use: Infuse 1 teaspoon of the dried flowers in 1 cup of boiling water for 15 minutes. Take 1 cup a day.

HOLLYHOCK

Botanical name: *Althaea rosea.*

Popular names: Garden hollyhock, common hollyhock.

Habitat: Cultivated.

Flora: Perennial, with mainly pink, yellow or red flowers August–October.

Folklore: The hollyhock was imported into Europe from China in the sixteenth century and soon became well established in English country gardens. Its medical uses were also quickly recognized by folk healers. The sixteenth-century herbalist William Turner, called it the holyoke (from which its common name derives), meaning 'holy plant', and it was also known popularly as beyond-the-sea, referring to its origins in the Far East. Hollyhocks have been used to produce a natural colourant for use in winemaking.

General medical properties: Antiphlogistic, emollient and laxative.

Specific properties: The hollyhock can be used to reduce internal and external inflammation, to stop bed-wetting and as a mouthwash for sore or bleeding gums.

Application and use: Infuse 1 teaspoon of the dried flowers in 1 cup of boiling water for 15 minutes. Take 1 cup a day, or use as a mouthwash as required.

HOP

Botanical name: *Humulus lupulus.*

Popular names: Hop bine, willow wolf.

Habitat: Wild in hedges, and cultivated.

Flora: Perennial, with green flowers in late summer.

Folklore: The common name is said to originate in the Old English *hopen* or *hoppan*, meaning 'to climb'. It derived its name of willow wolf from the habit of its leaves, which twined around willow trees in the wild. The hop is famous for its use in brewing beer; though it was known in the classical world for other attributes, in the medieval period it seems to have been cultivated only for this particular purpose. The oil from hops is used in perfume manufacture and its stem are used for basketwork. It is also a popular ingredient for herbal pillows, used in the Middle Ages as a sure cure for insomnia; scientific analysis of the hop has indicated that it does indeed contain certain effective sedatives. In the kitchen, the blanched leaves and buds can be eaten after boiling or steaming. Gerard recommended that the excess water from boiling hops should be added to the dough in breadmaking, to get rid of the lumps. Hop tea, widely used in folk medicine as a general tonic, was said to aid the digestion. A brown dye can be distilled from the leaves and flowers.

General medical properties: Sedative, tonic, diuretic, nervine and antibiotic.

Specific properties: Hops are generally recommended for treating insomnia and nervous disorders because they are a sedative. They also have a limited effect in cases of water retention.

Application and use: Infuse ½ oz of hops in 1 pint of boiling water. Cool, and take as required.

HOREHOUND
See White Horehound.

WHITE HOREHOUND

Botanical name: *Marrubium vulgare.*

Popular name: Hoarhound.

Habitat: Hedgerows and woodland.

Flora: Perennial, with white flowers June–July.

Folklore: Horehound is a bitter plant related to the various mints. Its common name comes from Old English *harhune*, meaning 'downy plant', and has nothing to do with dogs. Its botanical name is said to originate from a Hebrew word, *marob*, which means 'bitter juice'. It was one of the five bitter herbs which Jehova commanded the Israelites to eat during the Passover feast which celebrated their flight from Egyptian tyranny. Horehound has been used as a folk remedy for coughs for thousands of years and was known for this purpose in ancient Egypt. It is still included in some popular cough medicines sold over the chemist's counter in many European countries. Culpeper claims that horehound leaves made into an ointment, would stop skin growing over the nails. In the eighteenth century horehound was powdered and made into a snuff which, if mixed with salt, was said to be a cure for the bite of a mad dog.

General medical properties: Anti-catarrhal, expectorant, tonic, laxative and emmenagogue.

Specific properties: Horehound is principally used as an expectorant in the treatment of bronchitis, catarrh and persistent coughs. It can also be used to treat asthma, constipation, lung diseases and inhibited menstrual flow, and for easing childbirth. Externally, it can be applied to cuts, bruises and minor skin conditions.

Application and use:
Make a decoction of the dried flowers, seeds or juice as a remedy for poor breathing, coughs and lungs complaints: Infuse 1 oz of the leaves in boiling water, and sweeten with brown sugar or honey to conceal the bitter taste. Use also as a winter drink for sore throats. A syrup can be made by boiling 1 lb of brown sugar with 1 lb of leaves.

HORSE CHESTNUT

Botanical name: *Aesculus hippocastanum*.

Popular name: Conker tree.

Habitat: Woodland and roadsides.

Flora: Deciduous tree with white flowers in May and shiny brown fruit in green outer case September–October.

Folklore: In classical times the word *Aesculus* was used to denote oak trees, but the specific part of the horse chestnut's botanical name may derive from the fact that the fruit was used as cattle and horse feed. The tree was first imported into Europe from Asia as late as the sixteenth century. Its medical properties for easing the discomfort of piles soon became apparent to herbalists and folk healers. The nut-like fruits were carried as a charm against rheumatism by country people, but were said to be effective only if they had been stolen or obtained by begging.

General medical properties: Astringent, tonic, antirheumatic and antiphlogistic.

Specific properties: Horse chestnut fruits, or conkers as schoolchildren call them, are used in folk medicine as a tonic, to treat rheumatic pain, to thin the blood and to cure piles. The active ingredient is escin, medically recognized as an anti-inflammatory agent.

Application and use: *Use with caution, as large doses can be toxic, and only under the direction of a medical herbalist.*

HORSERADISH

Botanical name: *Armoracia rusticana.*

Popular names: Common or garden horseradish, red cole.

Habitat: Damp places and waysides, and cultivated.

Flora: Perennial, with white flowers June–September.

Folklore: Botanists believe that the botanical name is derived from an obscure Latin word meaning 'spoon' – a reference to the shape of the leaves – and a word meaning 'wild radish'. Gerard was responsible for its present name, although before his time it was called red cole. The plant does not seem to have been widely used for culinary purposes until the seventeenth century, after which, because of its popularity as a salad vegetable, its medical qualities too became well known.

General medical properties: Stimulant, diuretic, laxative and appetizer.

Specific properties: Horseradish is used in folk remedies to relieve the symptoms of colds, influenza, flatulence, fevers and urinary infection, and to increase the appetite. Externally, it can be used to treat chilblains and boils.

Application and use: Infuse 1 teaspoon of the powdered root in a cup of boiling water for 15 minutes. Take 1 cup a day. For chilblains and boils, apply slices of root direct to the painful area.

HORSETAIL

Botanical name: *Equisetum arvense.*

Popular names: Sharegrass, bottlebrush, pewterwort, shave-grass.

Habitat: Wet places and wasteland.

Flora: Perennial.

Folklore: Horsetail is a prolific plant, which once established on cultivated land is difficult to eradicate. One of the oldest species of plants, it first evolved in the earliest prehistoric period. Fossil remains suggest that the original horsetail was the size of a small tree. The Romans called it 'the herb of the earth' and ate it in salads. In the Middle Ages it was used for cleaning metal utensils and polishing wood and pewter, hence one of its popular names. It was also employed in cosmetics for strengthening fingernails.

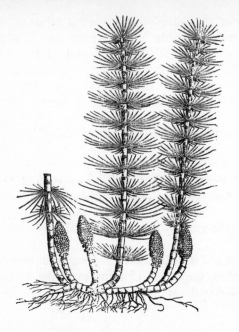

General medical properties: Diuretic, astringent, vulnerary and tonic.

Specific properties: Horsetail is used to treat kidney and bladder disorders, gastro-enteritis, the prostate gland and urinary infections. Externally it is applied to chilblains and open wounds.

Application and use: *Use with caution as it can cause internal irritation.* Steep 1 teaspoon of the leaves or whole plant in 1 cup of boiling water for 30 minutes. Take 1–3 cups a day. Apply the leaves externally as a poultice.

HOUNDSTONGUE

Botanical name: *Cynoglossum officinale.*

Popular names: Dog's tongue, gypsy flower, rats and mice.

Habitat: Wet places, wasteland and hedgerows.

Flora: Annual or biennial, with red-purple flowers May–September.

Folklore: As its common and popular names suggest, houndstongue was supposed to offer protection against attacks by savage dogs. The procedure was to wear a leaf from the plant in your shoe, and dogs would avoid you. Its leaves do in fact resemble a canine tongue. However, the plant also has an unpleasant smell reminiscent of mice, so in some country districts it was called rats and mice.

General medical properties: Demulcent, anti-inflammatory, anti-catarrhal and narcotic.

Specific properties: Houndstongue is recommended for soothing persistent coughs, treating lung diseases and for piles. The bruised leaves can be applied to relieve the discomfort of insect bites and stings. An ointment made from the leaves is said to cure baldness and will heal sores and ulcers.

Application and use: Steep 1 teaspoon of the dried root or leaves in 1 cup of boiling water. Take a sip at a time during the day.

KIDNEYWORT

Botanical name: *Anemone hepatica*.

Popular names: Liverwort, pennywort.

Habitat: Woodland, rocks and stone walls.

Flora: Perennial, with blue flowers in May.

Folklore: This plant derives its botanical name from Greek *hepataros*, 'liver', medieval herbalists used it to cure diseases of that organ. Culpeper assigned it to the planet Venus and the zodiac sign of Libra (23 September–22 October). According to him, the juice is favourable for 'unnatural heats' and curing 'St Anthony's fire' [sciatica]. Folk healers also recommended it for soothing the pain of gout.

General medical properties: Anti-inflammatory, diuretic, demulcent, tonic and expectorant.

Specific properties: Kidneywort can be used for water retention, bronchitis and kidney disorders. Externally it can be used to treat pimples, blemishes, boils, sores, sciatica, gout and swollen testicles.

Application and use: *Toxic if taken in large doses. Use only as directed by a medical herbalist.*

KNOTGRASS

Botanical name: *Polygonum aviculare.*

Popular Names: Birdweed, lowgrass, pigweed.

Habitat: Wasteland and fields.

Flora: Annual, with white flowers June–October.

Folklore: In his famous *Herbal* Culpeper says this plant is ruled by Saturn and comes under the zodiac sign of Capricorn (21 December–19 January). He recommended its use to stop blood flowing. The old herbalists regarded knotweed as a sure cure for the spitting of blood.

General medical properties: Astringent, coagulant, diuretic and expectorant.

Specific properties: Knotweed is suggested for treating dysentery, prolific menstrual flow, bronchitis, jaundice and lung disease. It is used particularly for dealing with internal bleeding, and can also dissolve kidney and gall bladder stones.

Application and use: Steep 3 teaspoons of the flowers in 1 cup of boiling water for 10 minutes. Take 1 cup a day.

LADY'S BEDSTRAW

Botanical name: *Galium verum.*

Popular names: Cheese rennet, yellow bedstraw, wild rosemary, maiden's hair.

Habitat: Meadows and hedgerows.

Flora: Perennial, with yellow and white flowers June–September.

Folklore: Lady's Bedstraw is very common all over the British Isles. Because of its pleasant, honey-like scent it was once used to stuff mattresses and as an insect repellent. Its popular name of cheese rennet indicates its use for curdling milk until the early nineteenth century; milkmaids also used the flowers to colour the milk used in cheese. In Gloucestershire it was used in making the distinctive deep yellow Double Gloucester cheese. In traditional folk remedies it is used as a nerve tonic and sedative.

General medical properties: Nervine, sedative, tonic, diuretic and insecticide.

Specific properties: Lady's bedstraw is used to treat hysteria, epilepsy and extreme nervousness. It also has limited use for skin diseases.

Application and use: Infuse 1 teaspoon of the flowers in 1 cup of boiling water for 15 minutes. Take 1 cup a day.

LADY'S MANTLE

Botanical name: *Alchemilla vulgaris.*

Popular name: Lion foot.

Habitat: Woodland and meadows.

Flora: Perennial, with greenish-yellow flowers May–June.

Folklore: The generic name means 'little magical one', and refers to the medieval belief that the plant had magical powers because of the fact that dew, an important ingredient in many medieval magical and alchemical rituals, gathers in its leaves overnight. Country people gathered this dew and used it as a beauty lotion. Culpeper claimed that women with sagging breasts could make them firm and rounded by smearing them with the juice of this plant. A pillow filled with the flowers was said to induce a good night's rest.

General medical properties: Sedative, anti-inflammatory, appetizer, astringent and tonic.

Specific properties: Lady's mantle was recommended by folk healers for treating inflammation, and it prevents excessive bleeding. It was much used in the past for what were called 'women's troubles' as it relieved the discomfort of the menopause and inhibited excessive menstruation. Externally, it heals sores and ulcers.

Application and use: Steep 1 teaspoon of the dried leaves in 1 cup of boiling water for 10 minutes. Take 1 cup a day.

LADY'S SMOCK

Botanical name: *Cardamine pratensis*.

Popular names: Cuckoo flower, bittercress.

Habitat: Fields, woodland and wet places.

Flora: Perennial with white flowers April–May.

Folklore: This plant, which is rich in vitamins, was once cultivated for use in salads as a substitute for watercress.

According to popular folk belief lady's smock was sacred to the fairies, and so it was considered very unlucky to bring it into the house because the fairies would be offended and seek revenge on the household. If the plant was included in May Day garlands the person carrying it would fall sick for the same reason.

General medical properties: Diuretic, appetizer, digestive and stomachic.

Specific properties: Lady's smock can be used to treat loss of appetite, indigestion, water retention and stomach upsets.

Application and use: Infuse 1 teaspoon of the fresh leaves or flowers in 1 cup of boiling water for 15 minutes. Take 1 cup a day.

LAVENDER

Botanical name: *Lavandula officinalis.*

Popular names: English lavender, garden lavender.

Habitat: Wild and cultivated.

Flora: Perennial, with purple flowers June–September.

Folklore: For centuries lavender has been used as a perfume, a sedative, a stimulant and for antiseptic purposes. The Romans used the plant in their bathwater and placed linen bags of it among their clothes as a natural deodorant. Its specific name is connected with the idea of washing. In the Middle Ages lavender oil was used to kill lice and bed bugs, while in warfare it was used as a natural antiseptic to cleanse sword cuts: modern scientists have discovered that lavender contains an essential oil which destroys bacteria on contact. In folk belief it is considered lucky to have a lavender bush growing in your garden, but the luck would vanish if flowers were cut and dried.

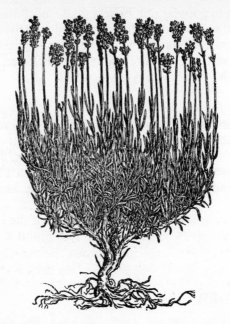

General medical properties: Antispasmodic, antibacterial, antiseptic, diuretic and sedative.

Specific properties: The principal use of the herb in folk remedies is for treating nervousness, insomnia, headaches and stress, and as a general antiseptic and pain reliever. It can also be used to treat rheumatism, depression, toothache, loss of voice, fainting and low blood pressure. Externally, it can be used to treat skin rashes and insect bites. It also acts as an insect repellent.

Application and use: Infuse 1 teaspoon of the dried herb in 1 cup of boiling water for 15 minutes. Take 3 times a day.

LILAC

Botanical name: *Syringa vulgaris.*

Popular name: Common or garden lilac.

Habitat: Cultivated.

Flora: Perennial, with white, pinkish-mauve or purple flowers in summer.

Folklore: Originally a native of Asia Minor, lilac was introduced into western Europe as a cultivated plant as late as the sixteenth century. Its original Persian name, *lilak*, was anglicized as lilac. Medically, the herbalists used it to treat fevers, as it was regarded as an alternative to quinine, which was very expensive. In folklore lilac is regarded as an unlucky flower to have inside the house because it is an omen of death.

General medical properties: Diuretic and anti-inflammatory.

Specific properties: Principally lilac is used for the treatment of fevers, especially in tropical diseases such as malaria. It has also been found of use in cases of rheumatism.

Application and use: Infuse 1 teaspoon of the leaves in 1 cup of boiling water for 15 minutes. Take 1 cup a day.

LILY OF THE VALLEY

Botanical name: *Convallaria majalis.*

Popular names: Wood lily, May lily, Our Lady's tears, May blossom.

Habitat: Dry woodlands, and cultivated.

Flora: Perennial, with white flowers May–June.

Folklore: As one of its popular names suggests, this plant was sacred to the Virgin Mary, who is the Christianized version of the old pagan Moon Goddess. Lily of the valley grew wild in the depths of St Leonard's Forest in Sussex, allegedly from the spots of blood shed during the saint's fight with a local dragon. The sweet smell of the flowers is said to be a powerful attraction to nightingales. Medieval herbalists used the plant as a substitute for foxglove, because it has a stimulating effect on the heart. In the First World War it was used to treat soldiers who had suffered the effects of mustard gas, as it has a strengthening effect on the nervous system.

General medical properties: Cardiac stimulant, diuretic, laxative and antispasmodic.

Specific properties: Recent research has revealed that lily of the valley contains a substance known as convallamarin, which is a potent cardiac stimulant similar to digitalis. This ingredient is now widely used by pharmaceutical companies in the manufacture of cardiac drugs. The flowers were believed to stimulate the mucous membranes of the nasal passages, and were recommended for treating sinusitis and vertigo. A spirit distilled from the flowers was applied externally for rheumatic pain. The traditional use of the plant is as a cardiotonic, but it also has a limited use in cases of water retention and nervous debility.

Application and use: *Only on the advice, and under the direction of, a medical herbalist.*

LIME TREE

Botanical name: *Tilia europea.*

Popular name: Linden.

Habitat: Cultivated.

Flora: Decidous tree, with yellow and white flowers at midsummer.

Folklore: The lime was a sacred tree to the ancient Teutonic peoples of northern Europe, possibly because, under ideal conditions, it can live for a thousand years. In popular folklore the tree was associated with death. At Cuckfield Hall in Sussex a famous lime tree stood for many years in the drive; everytime a branch fell from this old tree, a member of the family who lived in the house was said to die shortly afterwards. Medieval herbalists used a tea distilled from limeflowers to cure epilepsy; it was even said that an epileptic could be cured of their fits by just sitting under the tree. The bark of the tree was once used to make rope, and its wood was used in the manufacture of charcoal.

General medical properties: Antispasmodic, nervine, diuretic, expectorant and sedative.

Specific medical properties: Lime is recommended for the treatment of coughs, nervous disorders, hypertension, chills, fevers, migraine and catarrh, and externally as a soothing balm for skin rashes.

Application and use: Infuse 1 teaspoon of the fresh flowers in ½ cup of boiling water for 10 minutes. Take ½ cup a day.

LIQUORICE

Botanical name: *Glycyrrhiza glabra.*

Popular name: Liquorice.

Habitat: Cultivated.

Flora: Perennial, with lilac flowers June–July.

Folklore: The medical use of this plant dates back over three thousand years and is recorded in ancient Egyptian papyri. The ancient Greeks used liquorice as a thirst quencher, and children throughout the ages have eaten it as a confection. Liquorice grows wild in many parts of eastern Europe and Asia. It was first introduced into Europe in the fifteenth century, and brought to England by Dominican monks who grew it in their monastery garden at Pontefract in Yorkshire. Medieval herbalists used the plant as a natural sweetener to cover up the bitterness of other less palatable herbs in their compounds; it is some fifty times sweeter than sugar. Liquorice was also widely used as a cough medicine. In the 1940s a Dutchman, Dr F.E. Revers, discovered that his patients recovered more quickly from the effects of peptic ulcers if they took a herbal pill manufactured by a local pharmacist; when he analysed these pills he found that their main ingredient was liquorice.

General medical properties: Demulcent, anti-catarrhal, anti-spasmodic, laxative and anti-inflammatory.

Specific properties: Liquorice is used to treat bronchitis, coughs, gastric ulcers and indigestion, and externally as a wash for inflamed eyelids.

Application and use: Infuse 1 teaspoon of dried liquorice in 1 cup of boiling water for 15 minutes. Take 1 cup a day. *Overdosing can cause water retention.*

LOVAGE

Botanical name: *Levisticum officinale.*

Popular name: Sea parsley.

Habitat: Wet places, and cultivated.

Flora: Perennial, with whitish-yellow flowers July–September.

Folklore: Lovage derives its popular name from the fact that it was commonly eaten by sailors and fishermen as a cure for scurvy, caused by a lack of fresh vegetables; lovage contains an essential oil rich in vitamin C. The young leaves can be eaten raw in salads or cooked as a vegetable. The stems were once candied as a confection, and the root chewed as a tobacco substitute.

General medical properties: Diuretic and stimulant.

Specific properties: Lovage is recommended for use in cases of water retention and vitamin C deficiency.

Application and use: Infuse 1 teaspoon of the dried root or leaves in 1 cup of boiling water for 10 minutes. Take 1 cup a day.

LUNGWORT

Botanical name: *Pulmonaria officinalis*.

Popular names: Beggar's basket, Jerusalem cowslip, Jerusalem sage.

Habitat: Shady places and woodland.

Flora: Perennial, with pink and blue flowers March–May.

Folklore: The common name refers to the spotted leaves and the change in its flower colour from blue to pink, which resembled the symptoms of a diseased lung. For this reason lungwort was used in folk medicine to cure tuberculosis. Certainly its ingredients, such as tannin, silica and lime, can have a soothing effect on inflamed bronchial tubes.

General medical properties: Demulcent, expectorant, diuretic, astringent and anti-inflammatory.

Specific properties: The plant is recommended for the treatment of all lung diseases, bronchitis, coughs, catarrh and sore throats.

Application and use: Infuse 1 teaspoon of the dried herb in 1 cup of boiling water for 15 minutes. Take 1 cup a day.

MADDER

Botanical name: *Rubia peregrina*.

Popular name: Dyer's madder.

Habitat: Woodland and dry places, and cultivated.

Flora: Perennial, with greenish-yellow flowers June–September.

Folklore: As its common name suggests, madder was traditionally a source of a natural red dye called Turkey red or alizarin. Originally the plant was imported into Europe from Greece and Turkey as a commercial product for use by the linen industry. Until the end of the nineteenth century a compound of madder root, sheep's dung and alkali was used to dye wool and cotton; today it has been replaced by a synthetic substitute. In folk medicine madder root was used extensively to dissolve kidney stones.

General medical properties: Astringent, tonic, vulnerary, diuretic, laxative, antispasmodic and antiseptic.

Specific properties: Madder is used in the treatment of water retention, urinary infections and gall and kidney stones, and to cleanse open wounds.

Application and use: Infuse 1 teaspoon of the dried root in 1½ pints of boiling water in a closed container for 30 minutes. Cool and strain. Take 1–2 cups, cold, a day. Boil the root in honey and sugar to make a syrup. For removing skin blemishes, apply the bruised leaves externally.

MAIDENHAIR

Botanical name: *Adiantum capillus-veneris*.

Popular names: Venus hair, lady's hair.

Habitat: Wet places.

Flora: Perennial fern.

Folklore: Maidenhair derives its name from Greek *adiantos*, 'unwetted', because the foliage repels water and the plant generally is found in a damp environment. The popular folk names refer to the resemblance between the silky fronds of the fern and female pubic hair. Maidenhair was once a popular ingredient in a herbal cough medicine which was used until the end of the nineteenth century. Folk healers recommended its use in a herbal remedy to cure dandruff: the ashes of the burnt fern were added to vinegar and olive oil and then massaged into the scalp.

General medical properties: Expectorant, emmenagogue and diuretic.

Specific properties: Used in the treatment of asthma, bronchitis and water retention, and also to inhibit menstrual flow, dissolve kidney stones and purify the blood.

Application and use: Infuse 1 teaspoon of the fresh leaves in 1 cup of boiling water for 10 minutes. Take 1 cup daily.

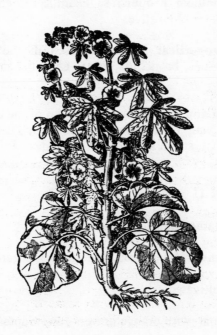

MALLOW

Botanical name: *Malva sylvestris.*

Popular name: Common mallow.

Habitat: Ditches and riverbanks.

Flora: Perennial, with pinkish-violet flowers June–September.

Folklore: Mallow has been cultivated since earliest times for both medicinal and culinary uses. In the sixteenth century the herbalists called it *Omnimorbia*, which means 'cure all', because of its superior powers. Its generic name, *Malva*, means 'soft', which refers to the texture of its leaves. Pliny the Elder, with his usual degree of exaggeration, claimed that anyone who took a spoonful of mallow would be instantly cured of any malady. Its leaves were once cooked as a vegetable and used raw in salads.

General medical properties: Demulcent, emollient, anti-inflammatory and laxative.

Specific properties: Mallow is used in the treatment of inflamed tissues, bronchitis, gastro-enteritis, sore throats and constipation.

Application and use: Infuse 1 teaspoon of the dried leaves or flowers in ½ cup of cold water for 8 hours. Then heat, but do not boil. Cool, strain and take ½ cup a day.

MARIGOLD

Botanical name: *Calendula officinalis.*

Popular names: Mary's gold, summer pride, garden marigold.

Habitat: Cultivated.

Flora: Annual, with orange flowers June–September.

Folklore: Marigold is a popular garden plant with an ancient history. It was known to the Romans, Greeks, ancient Egyptians, Arabs and Hindus. The generic name derives from Latin *calends*, 'throughout the months', a reference to the lengthy flowering season of the marigold. It was popularly called summer's pride, because it followed the sun and bloomed all through the hot weather. The plant has never been found in the wild and has only ever been cultivated. In folklore it is said that the flowers give off bright sparks during a thunderstorm. It was widely used in wedding bouquets because in flower symbolism it represents constant love. William Turner in his herbal says of the marigold, 'Some use it to make their hair yellow, not content with with the natural colour God has given them.' Rubbed on wasp stings, the flowers were said to bring instant relief. According to an old West Country belief, if you pick a bunch of marigolds at dawn you risk turning into an alcoholic. Welsh country folk say that if the blooms of marigold are not open by 7 a.m. there will be a thunderstorm by the end of the day. Marigolds were generally used in folk remedies as a natural antiseptic and to induce perspiration in fevers.

General medical properties: Astringent, antiseptic and anti-inflammatory.

Specific properties: Scientific tests with marigold have indicated that the plant lowers blood pressure and has a slight sedative effect. In folk medicine it is recommended for use externally to soothe burns, inflammation, skin rashes, irritated eyes and conjunctivitis.

Application and use: Infuse 2 teaspoons of the flowers in 1 cup of boiling water for 15 minutes. Take 3 times a day.

MARJORAM

Botanical name: *Origanum vulgare*.

Popular names: Wild marjoram, oregano, wintersweet, mountain mint.

Habitat: Dry grassland, and cultivated.

Flora: Perennial, with purple or pinkish-white flowers July–October.

Folklore: Marjoram is widely cultivated in western Europe but originated in the Mediterranean area. Its popular name of oregano comes from Greek *oros* and *ganos*, meaning 'joy of the mountain', because of the plant's attractive appearance. The ancient Greeks are reputed to have planted clumps of the herb over their tombs to give peace to the departed spirits and to stop them haunting the living. In folk belief marjoram seems to have been associated with fertility, because newly married couples were crowned with ringlets of the flowers. Today it is extensively cultivated for commercial use: as a herb it is used in meat dishes, and the oil has various uses in the cosmetic industry.

General medical properties: Expectorant, antiseptic, antispasmodic, anti-inflammatory, stomachic, nervine, appetizer, sedative and tonic.

Specific properties: As the list above indicates, this herb has many medical uses. It cleanses the body of impurities, purifies the bloodstream, cures yellow jaundice, stimulates the appetite, relieves deafness, eases toothache, calms nerves, cures stomach upsets, treats bronchitis and stops seasickness. Stuffed in a herbal pillow, the bruised leaves make a natural remedy for insomniacs.

Application and use: Infuse 2 teaspoons of the dried flowers in 1 cup of boiling water. Take 1–2 cups daily.

MARSHMALLOW

Botanical name: *Althaea officinalis.*

Popular name: Sweetweed.

Habitat: Wet places, ditches, riverbanks and cultivated.

Flora: Perennial, with white flowers July–September.

Folklore: This is another herb which has been cultivated for centuries. The Romans used it as a vegetable, the Greeks extolled its medical properties, and the Emperor Charlemagne promoted its use in Europe in the ninth century. Its most popular use is as a confection. During the Middle Ages folk healers recommended its use to treat various types of venereal diseases.

General medical properties: Demulcent and emollient.

Specific properties: When exposed to water marshmallow root swells to form a soothing gel; it therefore has wide uses in treating burns, skin diseases, rashes and cuts. The plant also reduces inflammation and has a pain-relieving effect on sore or cut skin. A poultice made of the ground root is effective for treating insect bites, and a wash made from the root or leaves can be used for dandruff or itchy scalps.

Application and use: Infuse 2 teaspoons of the dried leaves in 1 cup of boiling water for 10 minutes. Take 1 cup a day. Boil the flowers in water and strain off the liquid to use as a gargle. Dried root boiled in milk was an old folk remedy for whooping cough. For colds take 5 oz of flowers, 5 oz of dried root and 2 oz of raisins. Boil up in 5 pints of water until only 3 pints are left. Strain, and take ½ a wineglass a day until the symptoms ease.

MEADOWSWEET

Botanical name: *Filipendula ulmaria.*

Popular names: Queen of the meadow, bridewort, meadwort.

Habitat: Fields and meadows.

Flora: Perennial, with white flowers June–September.

Folklore: The original use of meadowsweet was as a flavouring agent in mead. In 1839 the flowers of the plant were found to contain salicylic acid, from which aspirin was synthesized. In folklore meadowsweet was associated with death, possibly because of its sweet-smelling flowers: its heavy scent was said to be able to induce a deep sleep from which the sleeper would never wake. For this reason it was never placed in bedrooms or sick rooms.

General medical properties: Antispasmodic, astringent, stomachic, anti-inflammatory and antirheumatic.

Specific properties: Meadowsweet can be used to prevent stomach disorders and for the treatment of heartburn, colic and peptic ulcers. It can also be used as an effective pain reliever for rheumatism, arthritis, fevers and chills.

Application and use: Infuse 1 teaspoon of the dried flowers or root stock in 1 cup of boiling water for 15 minutes. Take 1 cup a day.

MILKWORT

Botanical name: *Polygala vulgaris.*

Popular name: Rogation flower, gong flower, common milkwort.

Habitat: Meadows and hillsides.

Flora: Perennial, with blue flowers May–September.

Folklore: The generic name derives from Greek words meaning 'much milk', a reference to the milkwort's ability to increase the flow of breast milk in nursing mothers. Its other two popular names originated in its use in garlands carried by people following the old folk custom of Beating the Bounds.

General medical properties: Expectorant, diuretic, laxative, stomachic, appetizer and galactagogue.

Specific properties: As well as its common usage by mothers with new-born babies, milkwort was also recommended in folk remedies for treating coughs and stomach pains and for improving the appetite.

Application and use: Infuse 1 teaspoon of the dried root or plant in 1 cup of boiling water for 15 minutes. Take 1 cup a day.

MONEYWORT

Botanical name: *Lysimachia nummularia.*

Popular names: Herb twopence, creeping Jenny.

Habitat: Hedgerows and fields.

Flora: Perennial, with yellow flowers June–July.

Folklore: In his *Herbal* Culpeper places this plant astrologically under the rulership of the planet Venus and the goddess of love, for which reasons he recommends it for preventing the excessive flow of menstrual fluids. In folk medicine it was also used to curb internal bleeding.

General medical properties: Anticoagulant and stomachic.

Specific properties: As in the days of Culpeper, the primary use of this herb nowadays is for controlling menstruation and preventing internal haemorrhaging.

Application and use: Infuse 1 teaspoon of the dried herb in 1 cup of boiling water. Take 1 cup a day as required.

MOTHERWORT

Botanical name: *Leonurus cardiaca.*

Popular names: Lion's tail, throw wort.

Habitat: Rare, on wasteland and roadsides.

Flora: Perennial, with pink-purple flowers July–September.

Folklore: This plant was originally a native of central Asia. Its common name derives from its use by the ancient Greeks as a nerve tonic for pregnant woman, and it has been used in folk healing to cure infections of the vagina. The botanical name comes from Latin *leo*, 'lion', and Greek *oura*, 'tail', description of the leafy stem of the plant, with Greek *kardiaca*, 'heart', referring to its use in heart conditions. According to an old country saying, if you ate motherwort regularly you would 'live to be a source of continuous astonishment and grief to your waiting heirs'. So common was the belief that this herb had regenerative powers that it was sometimes called 'the herb of life'. Folk healers used it extensively for treating women suffering from menstruation problems and difficulties in childbirth. In the seventeenth century a distillation of motherwort was used to calm those suffering from epileptic fits. The plant was generally cultivated for its medicinal powers and was seldom found in the wild.

General medical properties: Sedative, nervine, anti-spasmodic, cardiac and tonic.

Specific properties: Medical tests indicate that extracts of this herb do have a tonic effect in some heart conditions. It has also been proved to have sedative and anti-epileptic properties. Motherwort is therefore recommended for treating female disorders, heart disease, hysteria, low blood pressure, extreme nervousness and palpitations.

Application and use: Infuse 1 teaspoon of the dried or fresh flowers in ½ cup of boiling water for 15 minutes. Take 1 cup a day.

MOUSE-EAR HAWKWEED

Botanical name: *Hieracium pilosella*.

Popular name: Mousewort.

Habitat: Wasteland, meadows and ditches.

Flora: Perennial, with yellow flowers in October.

Folklore: The name originates in the shape of the leaf which country folk thought resembled the shape of a mouse's ear, while 'Hawkweed' is a reference to the folk belief that hawks consumed the juice of this plant to increase their already considerable eyesight. For this reason medieval herbalists used extracts of the herb for treating eye diseases. In his *Herbal* Gerard claimed that it had the additional power of hardening metal! No scientific proof has been found to support his claim.

General medical properties: Expectorant, antispasmodic, anti-catarrhal, astringent, diuretic and anti-bacterial.

Specific properties: Mouse-ear hawkweed can be recommended for treating liver disorders, bronchitis, whooping cough and asthma, and as a natural antiseptic for open wounds.

MUGWORT

Botanical name: *Artemisia vulgaris.*

Popular names: Felon's herb, sailor's tobacco.

Habitat: Wasteland, hedgerows and banks.

Flora: Perennial, with yellow-red flowers July–October.

Folklore: Mugwort is a very ancient herb. Its common name dates from Anglo-Saxon times and is from Old English *muggia wort*, 'midge plant': it was evidently used to repel insects. Its generic name comes from the Greek goddess Artemis. Opinions differ among the experts as to why this plant became associated with this pagan Moon Goddess: most herbalists suggest it is because mugwort has proved successful in dealing with problems arising from the menstrual cycle, which is linked with the lunar phases; the Greeks also used the plant to ease difficult childbirth and to assist in the expelling of the placenta. Pliny the Elder suggested that all travellers should carry a sprig of Mugwort to prevent tiredness on a long journey. In 1656 William Coles, in his book *The Art of Simpling*, said that if a footman placed a mugwort leaf in his shoe he would be able to walk forty miles before noon without stopping or becoming tired. Mugwort leaves were placed under the pillows of sick people in the hope that they would be cured of their malady when they awoke. It was also an old country belief that a bunch of mugwort hung up in the kitchen would protect the house from lightning during a thunderstorm.

In the old days mugwort leaves were used to create a substance known as moxa. The dried leaves of the plant were bruised and rubbed between the hands until they became shredded; this substance was formed into a cone and placed upon the skin. It was then set alight and allowed to burn down until a blister was created on the skin. Incredibly this painful quasi-medical practice was still in use in France during the 1830s as a cure for a variety of diseases including asthma, rheumatism and paralysis of the limbs.

General medical properties: Nerve tonic, appetizer, laxative, sedative and emmenagogue.

Specific properties: Medical testing of this herb has indicated that it does stimulate uterine muscle, which would make it an effective treatment for inhibited menstruation. It has also been proved to have a limited sedative effect. Mugwort can be used as a tonic for nervousness, to ease tension and cure depression. It also helps to aid the normal flow of the menses, and its sedative properties have some use in treating epilepsy. Externally, it can be used to treat bruises and chilblains.

Application and use: Infuse 1 teaspoon of the dried leaves or flowers in 1½ cups of boiling water. Take 1 cup a day.

MULLEIN

Botanical name: *Verbascum thapsus.*

Popular names: Beggar's blanket, Adam's fennel, hare's beard, cow's lungwort, Aaron's rod, donkey's ears, candlewick, rabbit's ear, bull's ear, velvet dock, flannel dock, great mullein.

Habitat: Wasteland, woodland and hedgerows.

Flora: Perennial, with yellow flowers June–October.

Folklore: The common name of mullein comes from Latin *mollis*, 'soft'. This, like many of its popular names, is a reference to its large leaves, which have a velvety texture. Its folk name of candlewick dates back to the days when the stem was dried, dipped in tallow and used as a torch. Mullein leaves, greatly prized for decorative purposes, were included in herbal smoking mixtures and in the preparation of herbal cosmetics. In magical lore mullein was regarded as a herb of protection; it is even said that medieval monks grew it in their monastery gardens to ward off the Devil. In the Middle Ages the juice from the plant was used in folk remedies to cure gout and piles; the leaves and flowers were compounded, and then left to decay in a sealed wooden tub. After three months the juice was pressed out of the rotted plant material and corked in glass bottles ready for use.

General medical properties: Demulcent, expectorant, diuretic and sedative.

Specific properties: Mullein is recommended for treating bronchitis and asthma, as it has a beneficial effect on the respiratory system. Mullein leaves in hot vinegar and water can be applied to piles, and boiled with lard or vegetable fat they can be made into an ointment for dressing wounds. A poultice of the leaves or flowers can be applied to burns. Because of its unpleasant taste, mullein is sometimes best mixed with another herb.

Application and use: Infuse 1 teaspoon of the leaves or flowers in 1 cup of boiling water. Take ½ cup a day. Alternatively, boil 2 oz of leaves in 2 pints of water for 20 minutes. Drink the resulting liquid every 3 hours for severe bronchial congestion. Apply externally for swellings and itching, or use as a gargle.

NETTLE

Botanical name: *Urtica dioica.*

Popular name: Stinging nettle.

Habitat: Wasteland and roadsides.

Flora: Perennial.

Folklore: The common name of this well-known plant comes from an old word meaning 'to twist', and dates from the time when it was used to make fibre. In the past nettle was even cultivated for cloth manufacture. In ancient Greece it was used as an antidote for hemlock poisoning and as a cure for scorpion stings and snakebites. The medieval magician Albertus Magnus said that if you made an infusion of houseleek juice and nettles and rubbed it into your hands it would attract fish. In folklore, if you threw a bunch of nettle tops on the fire during a thunderstorm the house would be protected from lightning. A bunch of dried nettles hung in the larder warded off flies, and if hung near a hive drove away frogs. The popular phrase 'to grasp the nettle', meaning to take on an unpleasant task or face a difficult problem, originated in the folk belief that a person could be cured of a fever by pulling up a nettle with his or her bare hands.

The nettle is infamous because of the formic acid secreted by the hairs on the plant, which cause intense itching and skin blisters. Young nettles, before their stinging ability develops, have always been popular as a salad or an alternative to spinach. The plant is rich in vitamin A and C and various minerals, so is recommended for improving the complexion. Nettle seeds were once regarded as an aphrodisiac, and nettles were cultivated commercially as a source of chlorophyll.

General medical properties: Astringent, diuretic, appetizer, galactagogue and anti-coagulant.

Specific properties: Scientific tests have proved that nettle has the effect of lowering the blood sugar level, so it could have a use in treating diabetes. It can also be recommended as a stimulant to the appetite, a blood purifier and an aid to the digestion system; it lowers the blood pressure, increases the secretion of breast milk, can treat anaemia and stimulates the scalp in cases of premature baldness. Used as a snuff, the powdered leaf prevents nosebleeds and cures water retention.

Application and use: Only use fresh leaves, or cook them first. Infuse 2–3 tablespoons in 1 cup of boiling water and leave for 10 minutes. Take 1 tablespoon of the resulting liquid 4 times daily.

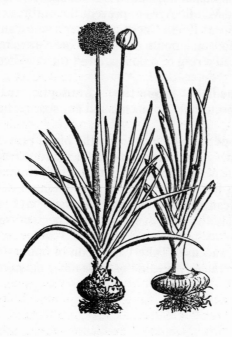

ONION

Botanical name: *Allium cepa*.

Popular name: Common onion.

Habitat: Cultivated.

Flora: Biennial or perennial, with whitish-green flowers June–August.

Folklore: The common onion has been cultivated as a food for thousands of years and is mentioned by the Assyrians, ancient Egyptians, Greeks and Romans. It is the most widely grown vegetable worldwide. In folklore it was claimed that onion seeds had to be sown on St Gregory's Day (12 March) to ensure a good crop. It was also believed that a raw onion would draw out the poison from a snakebite. Bunches of onions were hung outside houses in the Middle Ages to prevent the outbreak of bubonic plague. As late as 1968 a Cheshire farmer's wife claimed that an outbreak of foot and mouth disease had been prevented because she had placed a ring of onions around the cowshed.

General medical properties: Antiseptic, antibacterial, diuretic, expectorant, stomachic and antispasmodic.

Specific properties: Onions lower the blood pressure, restore sexual potency, promote urinary flow, and act as a natural antiseptic due to their sulphur content. Onion juice is known to be beneficial in the treatment of skin blemishes. Externally, onion juice can be used to treat chilblains and insect bites. Onions can also be used in syrups for persistent coughs.

Application and use: Take 1 teaspoon of onion juice 3 times daily. *Use with care, because in large doses the juice can be an irritant.*

PANSY

Botanical name: *Viola tricolor.*

Popular names: Stepmother, garden violet, heartsease, garden gate, love-in-idleness, Johnny-jump-in.

Habitat: Grassy places, and cultivated.

Flora: Annual, with purple, white and yellow flowers May–September.

Folklore: The common name pansy comes from the French *pensée*, meaning 'thought' or 'remembrance'. The white pansy flowers represented long thoughts, the yellow were souvenirs and the purple were memories, so a gift of pansies was used to ease the heartbreak between separated lovers. Folklore claims that to pick a pansy with dew on it will cause the death of a loved one; to pick pansies on a fine day will make it rain. Until about sixty years ago the pansy was cultivated in several European countries as a herbal treatment for heart disease.

General medical properties: Cathartic, demulcent, diuretic and anti-inflammatory.

Specific properties: Pansy is used in folk remedies as a safe and gentle laxative, for water retention, heart disease, hysteria and for easing childbirth. Externally, it can be used as a soothing balm for skin diseases.

Application and use: Infuse ½ oz of the flowers in 1 pint of water and steep for 15 minutes. Take 1–2 cups a day.

PARSLEY

Botanical name: *Petroselinum crispum*.

Popular name: Common parsley, garden parsley.

Habitat: Dry places, and cultivated.

Flora: Biennial and perennial, with whitish-green flowers June–August.

Folklore: Despite its common use as a culinary herb, parsley has always been regarded as an unlucky plant associated with death and funerals. The Romans believed that parsley had the power to make a pregnant woman miscarry, this may be the origin of the later folk belief that unwanted babies could be aborted if a woman ate a large quantity of parsley. It should be added that there is medical evidence to support this assertion. It was widely believed by country folk that parsley should never be transplanted or given away; it was even believed that if you mentioned a person's name while you were picking parsley he or she would sicken and die within seven days. Parsley was also said to have the magical power to weaken the structure of glass. A glass washed in parsley water would break, it was said, if only touched lightly. A green dye can be obtained from the stems, and the plant itself is a popular ingredient in sauces and garnish for fish dishes.

General medical properties: Antispasmodic, diuretic, expectorant, antiseptic and appetizer.

Specific properties: Parsley has a wide range of medical uses including the treatment of bronchitis, water retention, asthma and high blood pressure. It also helps the circulation; cleanses the kidneys and improves the appetite.

Application and use: Infuse 1 tablespoon of the dried herb in 1 cup of boiling water for 20 minutes. Take 1 cup a day. *Use with caution. Do not overdose. Not to be taken by pregnant women.*

PARSLEY PIERT

Botanical name: *Aphanes arvensis.*

Popular name: Breakstone parsley.

Habitat: Wasteland.

Flora: Annual, with green flowers May–October.

Folklore: The common name of this herb is derived from the French *perce pierre*, meaning a plant able to grow on common ground and which resembles parsley. Its popular name of breakstone parsley refers to its use by medieval herbalists to dissolve kidney and gall stones.

General medical properties: Diuretic and demulcent.

Specific properties: Used specifically to dissolve kidney and gall bladder stones and for the treatment of cystitis.

Application and use: Infuse 1 teaspoon of the dried herb in 1 cup of boiling water for 15 minutes. Take 1 cup a day.

PENNYROYAL

Botanical name: *Mentha pulegium.*

Popular names: Pudding grass, tickweed.

Habitat: Woodland and fields.

Flora: Perennial, with mauve flowers July–October.

Folklore: Pennyroyal belongs to the same family of plants as peppermint and spearmint. The name is a corruption of the French *puliol royale*, or royal thyme. Its specific name, *pulegium*, was given to the plant by Pliny the Elder and means 'flea': in Roman times pennyroyal was burnt to kill that insect.

General medical properties: Antispasmodic, stimulant, carminative and stomachic.

Specific properties: In medical tests pennyroyal has been proved to act as a stimulant to the uterus, and can therefore be used in any cases of suppressed menstruation. However, because of its toxic nature in large doses it has largely been superseded by peppermint for treating headaches, nervous tension and indigestion.

Application and use: *Only on the advice of a medical herbalist.*

PEPPERMINT

Botanical name: *Mentha × piperita*

Popular name: Mint.

Habitat: Cultivated.

Flora: Perennial, with mauve flowers July–October.

Folklore: Peppermint, one of the oldest cultivated herbs, was grown in ancient Egypt, used by the Greeks as a perfume, and employed by the Romans to flavour sauces and wine. Wealthy Roman noblewomen chewed peppermint leaves to stop bad breath. The leaves were also strewn in granaries in the ancient world to keep away rats and mice. Despite this long history, the use of peppermint in England is not recorded until the end of the seventeenth century, when a botanist saw it growing in a field in Hertfordshire and gave it the name by which it is now internationally well known. Today it is used in the manufacture of confectionery.

General medical properties: Antispasmodic, analgesic, nervine, carminative and appetizer.

Specific properties: Scientific tests have proved the use of peppermint as a muscle relaxant; for this reason it can be used to treat spasms and to relieve stomach cramps. It is also recommended for the relief of indigestion and flatulence and for promoting a healthy appetite. As in Roman times, it is recommended for the antisocial condition known as halitosis. Externally, it can be used to treat skin complaints.

Application and use: Infuse 2–3 teaspoons of the dried leaves in 1 cup of boiling water. Take 2 cups a day. *Do not prolong dosage any longer than 7 days.*

PERIWINKLE

Botanical names: *Vinca major, Vinca minor.*

Popular names: Greater and lesser periwinkle, sorcerer's violet, cut finger, blue buttons.

Habitat: Woodland, and cultivated.

Flora: Perennial, with pale blue flowers March–April.

Folklore: Periwinkle derived one of its popular names, cut finger, from its ability to stem bleeding. Sorcerer's violet comes from its use in medieval magic. Albertus Magnus says, in a grimoire or textbook written for aspiring magicians, 'Perrywinkle when it is beate into powdre with worms of ye earth wrapped around it names: *Vinca major, Vinca minor.*

Popular names: Greater and lesser periwinkle, sorcerer's violet, cut finger, blue buttons.

Habitat: Woodland, and cultivated.

Flora: Perennial, with uch in vogue in Victorian times, periwinkle represented virginity; it was also said to symbolize eternity, and for this reason was included in wreaths at the funerals of young children.

General medical properties: Astringent, sedative and anti-coagulant.

Specific properties: In the 1960s doctors extracted from the leaves of the tropical version of this plant a chemical which is used today in the treatment of leukaemia and Hodgkin's disease. The principal use of the English native species is to treat excessive bleeding, including menstruation. It can also be used in cases of dysentery, mouth ulcers, hysteria, epilepsy and bleeding gums caused by bad teeth.

Application and use: Infuse 1 teaspoon of the dried flowers in 1 cup of boiling water. Take 1 cup a day.

PINK

Botanical name: *Dianthus caryophyllus.*

Popular names: Gillyflower, old carnation, clove pink.

Habitat: Rocky places, and cultivated.

Flora: Perennial, with rose, purple or white flowers July–October.

Folklore: Gilly was the Old English name for July, referring to the month when the flower first appears. This traditional flower has been largely replaced by horticulturists with the more common carnation, which does not have the same potent scent. It is used commercially to flavour liqueurs and cordials.

General medical properties: Tonic, diuretic and anti-inflammatory.

Specific properties: Although it is seldom used by modern herbalists, pink can be recommended for soothing the symptoms of fever as it promotes perspiration and urine.

Application and use: Infuse 1 teaspoon of the dried flowers in 1 cup of boiling water for 15 minutes. Take 1 cup a day, as required.

PIMPERNEL

Botanical name: *Anagallis arvensis*.

Popular names: Poor man's weather glass, shepherd's barometer, laughter bringer, scarlet pimpernel.

Habitat: Fields and pastures.

Flora: Annual, with scarlet flowers May–September.

Folklore: The Greek name of this flower is a word meaning 'to delight'. Its popular name of laughter bringer also refers to the belief that this herb could cure depression. Traditionally, country people told the time by observing the flowers, which open in the morning and close in early afternoon – hence its other popular names. The flowers also close shortly before rain.

General medical properties: Diuretic.

Specific properties: Used for treating water retention and depression.

Application and use: *Only on the advice of a medical herbalist.*

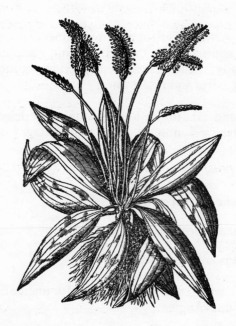

PLANTAIN

Botanical name: *Plantago major*.

Popular names: Greater plantain, ripplegrass, fireweed, rat tail, waybread, broadleaf, ribwort, lamb grass, lanceleaf, soldier's herb, ribgrass.

Habitat: Meadows and hedgerows.

Flora: Perennial, with white flowers April–November.

Folklore: Plantain has a long history in folk medicine for treating sores and ulcers. Country folk placed bruised leaves on open wounds as an emergency dressing: they believed it had the ability to close an open wound and heal it. Recently, medical tests have established that the plant contains a powerful antibacterial agent.

General medical properties: Demulcent, expectorant, vulnerary, diuretic, astringent and antibacterial.

Specific properties: This herb is recommended for treating bronchitis, coughs and sore throats, and for promoting urinary flow. Externally, the leaves can be applied in poultice form to treat wounds, sores and insect bites.

Application and use: Infuse 1 tablespoon of the dried leaves in ½ cup of water for 5 minutes. Take 1 cup a day.

POPPY

Botanical name: *Papaver rhoeas.*

Popular names: Corn poppy, Flanders poppy, opium poppy.

Habitat: Fields and hedgerows.

Flora: Annual with red flowers (*P. rhoeas*) or mauve flowers (*P. somniferum*) June–August.

Folklore: Poppies have been used as a colouring agent since at least the fifteenth century. A cough syrup made from the plant was employed by Arab physicians in the eleventh century. Country folk used to add poppy juice to their babies' bottles to get a good night's rest at teething time. Although the poppy is a source of the narcotic opium, it has also provided medical science with the greatest painkiller, morphine. The popular name of Flanders poppy refers to their widespread occurrence on the battlefields of the First World War.

General medical properties: Sedative, antihydrotic and antispasmodic.

Specific properties: Poppy promotes perspiration, soothes coughs and calms nervous restlessness. It is also good for treating anxiety attacks, hysteria, insomnia and fits.

Application and use: *Only on the direction of a medical herbalist.*

PRIMROSE

Botanical name: *Primula vulgaris.*

Popular name: Butter rose.

Habitat: Woods, hedgerows, roadsides and pastures.

Flora: Perennial, with yellow flowers April–June.

Folklore: Primrose comes from Latin *prima rosa*, 'first rose' (of the year), because it appears very early in the spring. According to folk belief it is very unlucky to bring a posy of these flowers into the house if they number fewer than thirteen plants. A smaller number indicates the number of eggs which the hens of the household will hatch that year. In magical lore primroses were used to protect barns and cowsheds from the evil spells of black witches. Children who eat primrose flowers are said to be able to see the fairies. In the New Forest wood cutters treated cuts with an ointment made of primrose oil boiled with lard. The flowers were also candied as a confection and used in salads.

General medical properties: Antispasmodic, expectorant and diuretic.

Specific properties: The principal use of primrose is to relieve lung congestion and treat bronchitis. It can also be used to ease childbirth and to treat pre-menstrual tension and nervous headaches. Externally, it reduces the swelling of bruises.

Application and use: Infuse 2 teaspoons of the dried flowers in ½ cup of boiling water. Take 1 cup a day.

PURPLE FLAG

Botanical name: *Iris versicolor*.

Popular names: Liver lily, flag lily, water flag, wild iris, fleur de lys.

Habitat: Wet places and cultivated.

Flora: Perennial, with blue or violet flowers June–August.

Folklore: One of this plant's popular names, liver lily, refers to its use in folk medicine to treat complaints of the liver. Folk healers also recommended its use for treating gastric disorders, as a blood purifier and for treating skin eruptions.

General medical properties: Diuretic, cathartic and alterative.

Specific properties: The root of the purple flag can be used to cure vomiting, heartburn, liver disorders, gall bladder infections and sinus problems. It is also widely used by folk healers and herbalists in the treatment of skin diseases, including eczema and psoriasis. It has a stimulating effect on the flow of saliva and the gastric juices. Externally, the bruised leaves relieve the swelling caused by bruises. *Use with caution, as large dosages can cause nausea.*

Application and use: Infuse 1 teaspoon of powdered root in 1 pint of boiling water. Cool, and take 2 tablespoons twice a day.

PURPLE LOOSESTRIFE

Botanical name: *Lythrum salicaria*.

Popular names: Grass Polly, willowherb.

Habitat: Riverbanks, ditches and wetlands.

Flora: Perennial, with purple flowers June–July.

Folklore: The botanical name is derived from Greek *lythrum*, 'blood', and *salaicaria*, 'willow', which refers to the shape of the leaves. In folklore loosestrife was said to have the power to calm wild animals, including horses. It was also popularly used as an insect repellent: in his *Herbal* Gerard says, 'The smoke of this burned herb driveth away serpents and kills gnats and flies in the house.' In magical lore loosestrife had the ability to encourage the development of psychic powers and restore the memory of past lives. The plant was once used commercially in tanning leather.

General medical properties: Astringent, antibacterial, tonic and antiseptic.

Specific properties: Widely used in folk medicine as an antiseptic for throat gargles and cleansing wounds.

Application and use: Infuse 1 teaspoon of the dried flowers in 1 cup of boiling water for 15 minutes. Take 1 cup a day.

RASPBERRY

Botanical name: *Rubus idaeus*.

Popular name: Wild raspberry.

Habitat: Shady places, and cultivated.

Flora: Perennial, with white flowers in spring and summer.

Folklore: Wild raspberries have been gathered since prehistoric times, but the cultivated variety was not introduced into Europe until the Middle Ages. In prehistoric times hunters used them as bait because bears loved them. Medieval folk healers used raspberry tea to cool fevers and as a proven cure for severe cases of insomnia.

General medical properties: Cardiac, laxative, galactagogue and astringent.

Specific properties: The astringent qualities of raspberry may be due to the high concentration of tannin in the leaves. The plant is believed to prevent vomiting, and is therefore recommended for treating morning sickness in pregnant women. It can also increase the secretion of breast milk, deaden labour pains, treat mouth ulcers, stop diarrhoea, act as a mouthwash for sore gums and mouth ulcers, and externally treat sores and cuts.

Application and use: Infuse 2 teaspoons of the fruit in 1 cup of boiling water for 15 minutes. Drink 1 cup as required.

RESTHARROW

Botanical name: *Ononis repens.*

Popular names: Cammock, stayplough.

Habitat: Meadows and pastures.

Flora: Perennial, with reddish-pink flowers.

Folklore: Restharrow is a pleasant-looking plant but should be treated with some respect as it possesses sharp spines. It also has a long root which makes it difficult to prise from the earth. Farmers called it stayplough, because the plant often became entangled around the plough and held it up. Not surprisingly, Culpeper placed this prickly plant under the dominion of the planet of war, Mars. In the Middle Ages folk healers used it to dissolve kidney and gall stones. They also mixed the powdered root with silver birch, meadowsweet and horsetail to make a herbal compound which promoted the flow of urine in cases of dropsy or water retention.

General medical properties: Laxative and diuretic.

Specific properties: Its principal uses are as a laxative, to treat water retention and to dissolve kidney and gall stones. It has some limited use for treating rheumatic pain, and externally for skin blemishes.

Application and use: Infuse 3–4 tablespoons of the root stock in 1 cup of boiling water for 15 minutes. Take 1 cup a day, lukewarm.

ROSEMARY

Botanical name: *Rosmarinus officinalis.*

Popular names: Rosa maria, dew-of-the-sea.

Habitat: Cultivated

Flora: Perennial, with pale blue flowers May–August.

Folklore: The plant's generic name translates from Latin as 'dew of the sea', this may be because the herb thrives near the sea. It was a sacred plant to the Romans, who burnt it as incense during religious ceremonies and planted it in wreath shapes for decorating the tombs of important people. The early Christian Church adopted rosemary as the sacred flower of the Virgin Mary. According to one legend, Mary sheltered under a rosemary bush with the baby Jesus during her flight to Egypt. Folk tradition states that, like the famous Glastonbury thorn, rosemary blooms at Christmas. Country people used branches of the plant to protect their homes from witches, evil spirits, fairies and lightning. A spring of rosemary placed under the pillow stopped nightmares, and it was even said that a comb made of the wood would cure baldness.

In an echo of the pagan Roman custom, bunches of rosemary were sometimes placed in the coffin at rural funerals. In the Middle Ages, folk belief credited rosemary with the ability of being an antidote to bubonic plague. A flourishing black market in the herb grew up, with one contemporary writer remarking that rosemary, which had been selling for 'twelve pence an armful', was being offered at 'six shillings a handful' when the plague broke out. Rosemary was also believed to be a protective plant which kept bad luck away, and a sprig placed in the buttonhole assisted business success and improved the memory. It was also used in love magic, for a sprig burnt slowly in a candle flame was said to be able to warm the heart of a cool lover. Oil of rosemary was first distilled in the fourteenth century and was extensively used in the manufacture of perfumes.

General medical properties: Tonic, diuretic, antispasmodic, stimulant, antiseptic, anti-depressive and appetizer.

Specific properties: Rosemary promotes regular liver function and can be used to treat neuralgia, high and low blood pressure, headaches, halitosis, depression, flatulence, premature baldness and loss of appetite; it also acts as a general tonic. Externally, it can be used to treat bruises and skin diseases, and it is an insect repellent.

Application and use: Infuse 1 teaspoon of the dried flowers in ½ cup of boiling water. Take one cup daily. *Use with caution.*

ROWAN

Botanical name: *Sorbus aucuparia.*

Popular names: Mountain ash, quicken tree.

Habitat: Woodland and gardens.

Flora: Perennial shrub or tree, with white flowers in May–June and red berries in autumn.

Folklore: Rowan was traditionally a tree which offered protection from the powers of darkness. Following Britain's conversion to Christianity this description usually referred to the old gods and goddesses who were worshipped in pagan times. Rowan twigs bound with red ribbons were hung over barn doors on May Eve (30 April) and Hallowe'en (31 October) to keep evil influences away from the livestock. Farmers' wives wore a necklace of dried rowan berries, to protect them from spells in case they met the local witch out walking. It was said that a plentiful crop of rowan berries signified a poor harvest the following season.

General medical properties: Aperient, astringent, diuretic and laxative.

Specific properties: Rowanberries can be used for water retention, as a purgative and as a gargle for sore throats.

Application and use: Take 1 teaspoon of rowanberry juice as required.

RUE

Botanical name: *Ruta graveolens.*

Popular name: Herb of grace.

Habitat: Cultivated and wild.

Flora: Perennial, with white and pink flowers July–September.

Folklore: Rue has always been regarded as an important plant, renowned for its medicinal and magical uses. The Romans claimed that eating it granted the gift of second sight or psychic vision. Musket balls soaked in rue water were said always to hit their target. The herb was also used for cursing rituals, but oddly was also said to be a protection against the evil spells of witches. The popular expression, 'You will rue the day . . .' originated in the folk belief that rue was a plant of misfortune. Traditionally rue was said, like rosemary, to be a powerful antidote to bubonic plague. In 1760 a rumour spread through London that the plague had broken out in St Thomas's Hospital: before the doctors at the hospital could issue a denial the price of rue in Covent Garden had doubled in price.

General medical properties: Antispasmodic, emmenagogue, nervine and stomachic.

Specific properties: The general use of rue is for treating stomach upsets and difficult menstruation, lowering blood pressure, easing nervous tension and relieving muscular cramps.

Application and use: *Use with caution. Over-dosing can cause abortions or skin allergies.* Infuse 1 teaspoon of dried herb in 1 cup of boiling water for 15 minutes. Take 1 cup a day, as required.

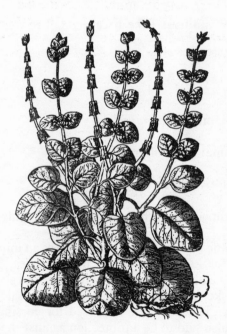

SAGE

Botanical name: *Salvia officinalis.*

Popular name: Garden sage.

Habitat: Cultivated.

Flora: Perennial, with purple, red, blue or white flowers June–July.

Folklore: Sage is a very ancient herb, whose generic name, *Salva*, means 'good health'. The Romans treated it as a sacred plant which had to be picked according to special religious rites: the gatherer had to wear a white robe, have bare feet and first indulge in a ritual bath; the plant also had to be gathered without using iron tools. Today we know that iron salts are incompatible with sage. According to the Roman belief a woman who cannot conceive should take sage juice, abstain from sexual intercourse for four days, and then go to bed with her husband. During the Middle Ages the herb was generally regarded as a cure-all. Culpeper said that it 'provoked the urine, expels the dead child, brings down women's courses and causes the hair to become black'. In folklore, it symbolized domestic virtue and was said to grow properly only in gardens where the wife ruled the household. Sage represented immortality, and eating it was said to rejuvenate the aged. In the old days a sprig of sage was hung in the kitchen when a member of the family was away; if it stayed fresh, the absent person was said to be happy. Eaten in May, the herb was said to be able to grant the eater a long and healthy life.

General medical properties: Antiseptic, anti-inflammatory, astringent and stomachic.

Specific properties: Sage reduces the flow of perspiration, treats dysentery, gastro-enteritis, sore throats and nervous disorders, and applied externally eases insect bites.

Application and use: Infuse 1 teaspoon of the leaves in ½ cup of boiling water for 30 minutes. Take 1 cup a day, a tablespoon at a time.

SAVORY

Botanical name: *Satureja hortensis*.

Popular names: Summer savory, garden savory.

Habitat: Cultivated.

Flora: Annual, with rose and lilac flowers August–October.

Folklore: Savory has been cultivated since the ninth century as a culinary herb, although its use as a medicinal plant dates back nearly two thousand years. It was renowned as an aphrodisiac, as indicated by its generic name, *Satureja*, which originated in the Greek word for a satyr, a lusty wood spirit. The Roman poet Virgil recommended that the herb should be planted around hives to attract bees. As a culinary herb savory is added to salads, sauces and vegetables. It is especially used on the Continent with haricot beans, hence its German name of *Bohnenkraut* or 'bean herb'.

General medical properties: Antiseptic, expectorant, carminative, stomachic, stimulant, diuretic and appetizer.

Specific properties: The principal use of savory is to stimulate the appetite and treat gastric complaints. It can also be used as an antiseptic gargle for sore throats and mouth ulcers.

Application and use: Infuse 2–4 teaspoons of the dried leaves in 1 cup of boiling water Take 1 cup a day.

SELF HEAL

Botanical name: *Prunella vulgaris*.

Popular names: Healwort, woundwort, heal all, sicklewort.

Habitat: Woodlands and pastures.

Flora: Perennial, with violet or purple flowers June–September.

Folklore: As its name suggests, self heal has a long history as a medicinal plant. Medieval herbalists who ascribed to the Doctrine of Signatures saw a resemblance between this plant and the throat, for which reason it was often included in folk remedies which treated this part of the body. The generic name is derived from a German word for quinsy, *Bräune*.

General medical properties: Astringent, tonic, antiseptic and carminative.

Specific properties: It is used to treat diphtheria, mouth ulcers, sore throats and burns.

Application and use: Infuse 2 teaspoons of the dried leaves for 15 minutes in 1 cup of boiling water. Take 1 cup a day, or use as a gargle as required.

SHEPHERD'S PURSE

Botanical name: *Capsella bursa-pastoris.*

Popular names: Shovelweed, St James' weed, toywort.

Habitat: Woodland and old ruins.

Flora: Annual or biennial with white flowers throughout the summer.

Folklore: The botanical name means 'the little case of the shepherd', a reference to its small triangular seedcases which resemble the purses once commonly worn by shepherds on their belts. Shepherd's purse grows as far north as Greenland, where it was introduced by the Vikings over a thousand years ago.

General medical properties: Anti-haemorrhagic, diuretic, emmenagogue, anti-inflammatory and astringent.

Specific properties: This herb is recommended for treating kidney disorders, low blood pressure, diarrhoea, wounds and nosebleeds, and for stimulating menstrual flow. Externally, it reduces the inflammation of chilblains.

Application and use: Infuse 2 teaspoons of the dried flowers in ½ cup of boiling water. Take 1 cup a day.

SKULLCAP

Botanical name: *Scutellaria galericulata*.

Popular names: Mad dog, mad weed, hooded willow herb.

Habitat: Wet places, ditches and riverbanks.

Flora: Perennial, with pale blue or purple flowers July–September.

Folklore: In the eighteenth century herbalists recommended this plant to treat rabies, hence its popular name of mad dog. It was also used to treat nervous tremors, lockjaw and convulsions. Its common name of skullcap refers to its use for mental patients.

General medical properties: Tonic, nervine, sedative and antispasmodic.

Specific properties: Skullcap is used principally to treat nervous disorders, insomnia, pre-menstrual tension, hysteria, muscular spasms and high blood pressure.

Application and use: Use with caution as can cause drowsiness. Infuse 1 teaspoon of the dried herbs in 1 cup of boiling water for 20–30 minutes. Take 2–3 times a day.

SLIPPERY ELM

Botanical name: *Ulmus fulva*.

Popular names: Red elm, sweet elm.

Habitat: Woodland.

Flora: Deciduous tree.

Folklore: This tree takes its name from the moist inner bark, which in powdered form is a very effective laxative and aid to childbirth. It is widely available as a commercial product in health food stores.

General medical properties: Demulcent, emollient and purgative.

Specific properties: Slippery elm can be used internally as a safe laxative for constipation, and externally for treating boils.

Application and use: Decoct 1 part of powdered bark to 8 parts of water. Boil, and simmer slowly for 15 minutes. Take ½ cup a day.

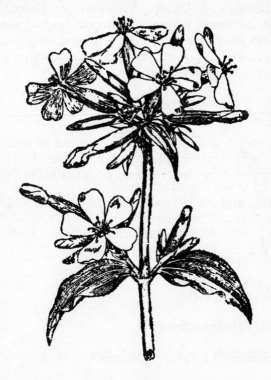

SOAPWORT

Botanical name: *Saponaria officinalis.*

Popular names: Bouncing Bet, fuller's herb, bruisewort, sheepweed.

Habitat: Wasteland and roadsides.

Flora: Perennial, with pink or white flowers June–September.

Folklore: The common name derives from the fact that in water the root exudes a substance known as saponin which creates a lather similar to soap. The detergent effects led to the plant's use as a natural alternative for soap, especially in the cleansing of wool before dyeing. The popular name of fuller's herb is a reference to the fullers who worked in the weaving industry. In 1548, in his book *The Names of Herbs*, William Turner first gave this plant its name of soapwort. However, it was known earlier to the Arab physicians, who used it to treat leprosy and other serious skin diseases. Medieval herbalists recommended soapwort for treating skin blemishes.

General medical properties: Antirheumatic, diuretic, depurative and expectorant.

Specific properties: Soapwort can be used to treat exzema, psoriasis, acne, scabies and other skin diseases. It also acts as a blood purifier, cures water retention and calms bad coughs.

Application and use: *Use only as directed by a medical herbalist.*

SORREL
See Wood Sorrel.

SOUTHERNWOOD

Botanical: *Artemisia abrotanum.*

Popular names: Lad's love, old man.

Habitat: Wild, and cultivated

Flora: Perennial, with yellowish-white flowers July–September.

Folklore: The common name originated in the Old English word *suthernwuld*, meaning 'a wooded plant from the south', a reference to its botanical origins in southern Europe. Because it is a strong-smelling herb it was formerly used to repel insects and as a nosegay to be carried by wealthy people to disguise the nastier smells of the streets. Medieval herbalists thought the herb had aphroidisiac powers, hence its name lad's love.

General medical properties: Stimulant, insecticide, antiseptic and emmenagogue.

Specific properties: It is principally used to promote menstruation in difficult cases, and as a general herbal antiseptic.

Application and use: Infuse 1 teaspoon of the dried herb in boiling water for 15 minutes. Take 1 cup a day.

SPEARMINT

Botanical name: *Mentha spicata*.

Popular name: Mint.

Habitat: Cultivated.

Flora: Perennial, with purple flowers July–September.

Folklore: Spearmint was introduced into Europe by the Romans, although its name dates only from the sixteenth century. Today, like peppermint, it is widely used as an essential oil for making confectionery. Spearmint has a sweeter, smoother taste than peppermint, which can be harsh. Folk healers used spearmint to cover the taste of unpleasant herbs in their remedies, or on its own as an aid to digestion.

General medical properties: Antispasmodic, digestive, stimulant and diuretic.

Specific properties: Spearmint is generally used in folk remedies to cure indigestion, flatulence, cramp, headaches, and colds.

Application and use: Infuse 1 teaspoon of the leaves in 1 cup of boiling water for 15 minutes. Take 1 cup a day.

SPEEDWELL

Botanical name: *Veronica officinalis.*

Popular names: St Llewellyn herb, gypsyweed, bird's eye, cat's eye.

Habitat: Hedgerows, woodland and heaths.

Flora: Perennial, with pale blue flowers May–August.

Folklore: This herb, as its common name suggests, was widely praised by folk healers for its fast-working curative powers. It was generally used in folk remedies for curing skin diseases and for both stomach and respiratory problems. In several European countries, including France and Germany, it was used as a substitute for tea.

General medical properties: Expectorant, stomachic, diuretic and appetizer.

Specific properties: Today the medicinal qualities of speedwell are treated with some scepticism by most herbalists. It is generally used in herbal tea mixtures, but can also be used to treat bronchitis, water retention and stomach upsets.

Application and use: Infuse 2 teaspoons of the dried flowers in ½ cup of boiling water. Take 1 cup a day.

ST JOHN'S WORT

Botanical name: *Hypericum perforatum*.

Popular name: Fairy herb.

Habitat: Woodland and meadows.

Flora: Perennial, with yellow flowers June–October.

Folklore: St John's wort derives its generic name of *Hypericum* from the Greek, which indicated that it smelt strong enough to drive away evil influences. It has always been recognized in folk belief as a plant which had the power to drive away witches, ghosts and demons. It could also protect a house from lightning. One Latin name for the herb used by medieval herbalists was *Euga daemonum*, or 'flight of demons'. Its common name derives from the fact that it is in full bloom at midsummer, which coincides with the Christian feast day of St John (24 June). Culpeper recommended a tincture of the flowers in spirits of wine to ward of melancholy and insanity. In the Doctrine of Signatures the red juice of the plant, which resembles blood, led to its use to treat open wounds. The popular name of fairy herb may refer to the belief on the Isle of Man that anyone who stepped on this plant would be carried off by the little people.

General medical properties: Diuretic, sedative, anti-inflammatory, astringent and anti-depressant.

Specific properties: *St John's wort has been found to contain a phototoxic agent which can react on fair-skinned people who are sensitive to sunlight. It should therefore only be used externally to treat skin irritations and insect bites.*

Application and use: *Only on the advice of a medical herbalist.*

STRAWBERRY

Botanical name: *Fragaria vesca*.

Popular names: Wild strawberry, wood strawberry.

Habitat: Grass and woodland, and cultivated.

Flora: Perennial, with white flowers May–June followed by red fruits.

Folklore: Although the strawberry has been cultivated since the sixteenth century in England as a dessert fruit, it was used for centuries before as a medicinal plant. Because of its high iron content strawberry has been recommended for people suffering from anaemia. It has also shown beneficial effects on the kidneys as well as lowering high blood pressure and treating gastro-enteritis. Externally, crushed strawberries have been used by women as a face pack to cleanse the complexion. Strawberries rubbed on chilblains are said to ease the severe itching sensation. It also has a use as a general tonic for children and sick adults, and many orthodox pharmaceutical products use strawberry syrup as a base.

General medical properties: Astringent, tonic, laxative and diuretic.

Specific properties: Strawberries are recommended as a gentle laxative, for water retention and as a tonic.

Application and use: Infuse the fruit in boiling water and take as required. *Caution: strawberries can cause allergic reactions in some people.*

SWEET FLAG

Botanical name: *Acorus calamus*.

Popular names: Sweet sedge, myrtle, sweet root.

Habitat: Wet places, riverbanks and ditches.

Flora: Perennial, with greenish-yellow flowers May–June.

Folklore: This ancient herb is mentioned in the biblical book of Exodus. It was introduced into Russia by the Mongols in the eleventh century, and from there to Poland in the thirteenth century; by the end of the sixteenth century it was widely distributed all over Europe. The medical properties of the root were well known to the ancient Greek and Arab physicians who used it as an aid to digestion, for expelling worms and for the treatment of colic.

General medical properties: Carminative, sedative and appetizer.

Specific properties: The general use of the root is in the treatment of severe cases of colic and flatulence. It has also been given as a sedative for the nervous system and as an appetite improver.

Application and use: Infuse 1 teaspoon of the dried root in 1½ pints of water. Drink 1–2 cups a day, lukewarm, as required.

SWEET VIOLET

Botanical name: *Viola odorata.*

Popular name: Sweet violet.

Habitat: Woodlands and hedges, and cultivated.

Flora: Perennial, with violet flowers April–May.

Folklore: This plant has been used in perfumery for nearly two thousand years. In the nineteenth century violet water was the most popular perfume used by ladies of distinction. It has also been used as a colouring agent for soft drinks and confectionery. Sweet violet also has important medical properties.

General medical properties: Purgative, expectorant and diuretic.

Specific properties: Sweet violet is recommended for treating bronchitis, catarrh and asthma. It can also be used as a laxative and to treat water retention.

Application and use: Infuse 1 teaspoon of the dried herb in 1 cup of boiling water for 10 minutes. Take 1 cup a day, as required.

TANSY

Botanical name: *Tanacetum vulgare*.

Popular names: Bitter button, wormwort, parsley fern.

Habitat: Woodland and wasteland.

Flora: Perennial, with yellow flowers July–September.

Folklore: Tansy was once used extensively to treat parasitic worms. In ancient times tansy oil was smeared on corpses, or bunches of it were placed in the shrouds of the dead, to keep away maggots. In the Middle Ages the herb was strewn on cottage floors to repel insects; it was also rubbed over meat to keep flies away. In the eighteenth century its bitter juice was used to flavour special cakes eaten at Lent; the idea was that the bitterness would remind the eater of the agonies suffered by Jesus on the cross. According to the old rhyme,

> On Easter Sunday is the pudding seen
> To which the Tansy lends her sober green.

General medical properties: Vermifuge, carminative, insectide and digestive.

Specific properties: The principal use of this herb is for expelling worms, but it should be taken with caution. Externally, it can be used to treat skin diseases and bruises.

Application and use: *Use only on the advice of a medical herbalist.*

TARRAGON

Botanical name: *Artemisia dracunculus*.

Popular name: French tarragon.

Habitat: Cultivated.

Flora: Perennial, with lilac or white flowers June–September.

Folklore: This herb is generally used to flavour chicken, seafood and meat. As its popular name suggests, it was widely used in French cuisine. Originally a native of Siberia, this herb has a number of medical uses.

General medical properties: Stomachic, digestive, diuretic and appetizer.

Specific properties: Tarragon is used for treating colic, flatulence, indigestion and nausea. It also has the ability to improve the appetite.

Application and use: Infuse ½ teaspoon of the dried herb in ½ cup of boiling water. Take ½ cup 3 times daily.

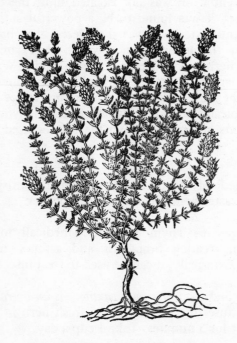

THYME

Botanical name: *Thymus vulgaris.*

Popular names: Common thyme, garden thyme.

Habitat: Cultivated.

Flora: Perennial, with lilac or white flowers June–September.

Folklore: According to legend, this plant grew from the tears shed by the beautiful Helen of Troy. The ancient Egyptians used it in the compound they mixed to embalm their dead. Opinions differ as to when it was first introduced into the British Isles: some botanists claim that the Romans introduced it, while others say that it did not arrive until the ninth century. Thyme's essential oil was not isolated until the eighteenth century, when it was found to be a powerful antiseptic. In modern scientific tests it was discovered that bacteria are destroyed by thyme oil essence within thirty minutes. In folklore this herb is associated with death, and in Wales it was often seen planted on graves. Thyme was also linked in folk belief with the fairies: a seventeenth-century recipe preserved in the Ashmolean Museum in Oxford mentions thyme as one of the ingredients of a magical elixir that can be used to see the little people.

General medical properties: Antiseptic, antispasmodic, expectorant, astringent, digestive and appetizer.

Specific properties: Thyme can be used medically for soothing sore throats, treating bronchitis and asthma and easing indigestion. Externally, it can be used to treat insect bites.

Application and use: *Use with caution, as an overdose can be poisonous.* Infuse ½ teaspoon of the fresh herb in ½ cup of boiling water for 5 minutes. Take 1 cup a day.

VALERIAN

Botanical name: *Valeriana officinalis*.

Popular names: Common valerian, all heal.

Habitat: Meadows, riversides and ditches.

Flora: Perennial, with white and pinkish flowers June–September.

Folklore: Valerian, named in the tenth century, was much sought after by Arab physicians. It has been described as the perfect herbal tranquillizer, and was used for this purpose in the First World War to treat soldiers suffering from shell shock. In the Middle Ages it was widely used by folk healers to treat the symptoms of epilepsy. The herb attracts rats, and it has been suggested that the secret weapon used by the Pied Piper of Hamelin may have been sprigs of valerian. In English folklore this herb was reputed to have aphrodisiac qualities: a young woman who carried a sprig of this herb was said never to lack ardent lovers. It was also said to possess the ability to increase psychic perception.

General medical properties: Sedative, antispasmodic, nervine and stomachic.

Specific properties: Medical tests have revealed that the roots of this plant contain substances known as valepotriates, which have a sedative effect. It is principally used in folk medicine to treat nervous tension, hyperactivity and insomnia, and as a general nerve tonic and sedative. As a pain reliever it can be recommended for severe headaches and rheumatic pains.

Application and use: Infuse 1 teaspoon of the dried root in 1 cup of boiling water for 15 minutes. Take 1 cup a day.

VERVAIN

Botanical name: *Verbena officinalis*.

Popular names: Simpler's joy, holy herb.

Habitat: Hedgerows and wasteland.

Flora: Perennial, with lilac flowers July–October.

Folklore: Vervain has an ancient history as a magical plant dating back to Greek times. The Romans called it *Herba Veneris* because they regarded it as sacred to the goddess of love, Venus. The Celtic druids were said to have washed their stone altars with water made from this herb before offering sacrifices to their gods. Country folk gathered the herb at specific phases of the moon and wore it as a protection against black magic. It allegedly possessed the mystical power of opening locked doors, and so was much valued by burglars. Hung around the neck, it was said to drive away bad dreams. In the Middle Ages the plant was used in love potions by white witches. Medically, vervain was used in folk remedies to cleanse the body of impurities, and was regarded as an antidote to poison and a cure for the bites of mad dogs and snakes.

General medical propertes: Tonic, astringent, diuretic and antispasmodic.

Specific properties: Vervain is recommended for treating disorders of the nervous system, depression, stress, hysteria, anaemia, pre-menstrual tension and muscular spasms. It can also be used to treat inflammation of the gall bladder and sore gums. Externally, an ointment made from the herb cures piles.

Application and use: Infuse 2 teaspoons of the dried herb in 1 cup of boiling water for 15 minutes. Take 1 cup a day.

VIOLET

See Sweet Violet.

WATERCRESS

Botanical name: *Nasturtium officinale.*

Popular name: Common watercress.

Habitat: Wet places, and cultivated.

Flora: Perennial aquatic, with white flowers June–September.

Folklore: Watercress is such a popular summer salad ingredient that its medical properties have largely been ignored. Its generic name means 'distortion of the nose', and refers to its pungent smell, caused by the high iron content. Medieval herbalists recommended people to wash their hair in watercress water to stimulate its growth.

General medical properties: Diuretic, stimulant, stomachic and expectorant.

Specific properties: It is recommended for treating anaemia (because of its high iron content), nervousness, bronchitis, asthma, urinary infection, water retention, diabetes, vitamin C deficiency and lack of appetite. Externally, it treats chilblains.

Application and use: *Use with caution, as prolonged dosage at high levels can cause kidney problems.* Infuse 1 teaspoon of young shoots in ½ cup of cold water. Do not boil. Take 1 cup 3 times a day.

WHITE BRYONY

Botanical name: *Bryonia dioica.*

Popular names: Ladies' seal, mandragora, English mandrake, devil's turnip, wild vine.

Habitat: Woodland and hedgerows.

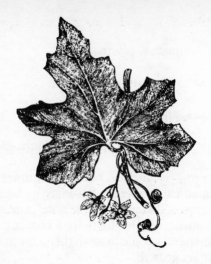

Flora: Perennial, with greenish-white or pale green star-shaped flowers with five petals. The root resembles a large turnip in shape and is yellowish-grey on the outside and white inside. The berries are red.

Folklore: The name Bryony is derived from the Greek word *bruein*, meaning 'to grow luxuriantly'. In the Middle Ages white bryony was the English equivalent of mandrake, used for magical purposes on the Continent, and was therefore much sought after by witches, magicians, alchemists and other practitioners of the occult arts. Bryony roots carved into the shape of human forms were used as shop signs by eighteenth-century herbalists. The plant was popularly regarded as having aphrodisiac properties, but this has never been proved. The ancient Romans regarded it as a protection against lightning: the Emperor Augustus Caesar always wore a wreath of bryony leaves on his head during thunderstorms. White bryony is not related to black bryony, *Tamus communis*.

General medical properties: Hydrogogue and cathartic.

Specific properties: The dried root is the part used in folk remedies. *However it is toxic and can cause vomiting and gastric pains; both berries and root are poisonous.*

Application and use: *Only under the direction of a medical herbalist.*

WINTERGREEN

Botanical name: *Pyrola minor.*

Popular names: Spice berry, mountain tea, deerberry.

Habitat: Woodland, and damp and hilly places.

Flora: Evergreen, with white flowers June–September.

Folklore: The principal ingredient of this important medical plant is methyl salicylate, which is the basis of opium! For this reason wintergreen has been used in folk remedies to alleviate pain.

General medical properties: Astringent, demulcent, diuretic and tonic.

Specific properties: Oil of wintergreen is recommended for soothing all forms of pain, including rheumatic, arthritis and migraine. It can also be used as a gargle, and externally to treat bruises.

Application and use: Infuse 1 teaspoon of the leaves in 1 cup of boiling water for 15 minutes. Take 1 cup a day.

WITCH HAZEL

Botanical name: *Hamamelis virginiana.*

Popular names: Spotted hazel, winterbloom.

Habitat: Woodland and gardens.

Flora: Tree or shrub, with yellow flowers September–October.

Folklore: Witch hazel is commercially produced for a liniment to treat bruises and cuts. The North American Indians used its branches as divining rods to find water.

General medical properties: Astringent and anti-inflammatory.

Specific properties: Witch hazel can be used to stop bleeding and to treat boils, insect bites, swellings, bruises, burns and cuts.

Application and use: Infuse 1 teaspoon of the dried leaves in 1 cup of boiling water for 15 minutes. Take 1 cup a day as required.

WOODRUFF

Botanical name: *Galium odoratum.*

Popular names: Sweet woodruff, Waldmeister's tea.

Habitat: Woodland and hedgerows.

Flora: Perennial, with white flowers May–June.

Folklore: Woodruff was renowned for its fragrance, and in the Middle Ages its flowers were strewn on the floors of houses and churches. Bundles of the herb were hung in houses during the summer to cool and freshen the air; it was also placed in wardrobes to scent linen and ward off moths. In some European countries the plant is distilled into a fragrant wine which is sold as a herb tonic.

General medical properties: Carminative, diuretic, tonic, stomachic and cardiac.

Specific properties: Woodruff is used for the relief of stomach pains, as a heart tonic and a cure for insomnia, and for liver and kidney disorders.

Application and use: *Only under the direction of a medical herbalist.*

WOOD SORREL

Botanical name: *Oxalis acetosella.*

Popular name: Irish shamrock.

Habitat: Woodland.

Flora: Perennial, with white flowers May–June.

Folklore: The generic name comes from Greek *oxalis*, 'sour'. The principal ingredient of wood sorrel is oxalic acid, which if taken in excess can cause the formation of kidney stones. The plant has been cultivated as a culinary herb for sauces since the fourteenth century, but has now largely been replaced by common sorrel, which is of French origin.

General medical properties: Diuretic and antiseptic.

Specific properties: It is used as a gargle, and externally for treating skin diseases.

Application and use: *Only on the advice of a medical herbalist.*

WORMWOOD

Botanical name: *Artemisia absinthium.*

Popular name: Absinthe.

Habitat: Waste places, and cultivated.

Flora: Perennial, with yellow-green flowers July–October.

Folklore: As its common name suggests this herb was extensively used in folk remedies to expel worms. Because of its

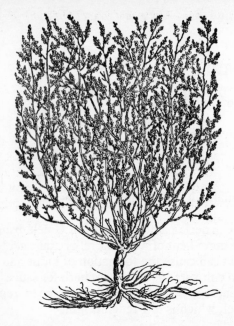

bitterness it has also been used commercially in the production of various aperitifs; absinthe itself had very dangerous side-effects, including hallucinations and brain damage. Medieval herbalists recommended this herb for treating water retention and as an antidote to poison.

General medical properties: Antiseptic, astringent and diuretic.

Specific properties: It is used for treating worms and as an appetizer.

Application and use: *Only on the advice of a medical herbalist. An overdose causes severe vomiting.*

YARROW

Botanical name: *Achillea millefolium.*

Popular names: Milfoil, woundwort, carpenter's weed, devil's plaything, nosebleed.

Habitat: Pastureland.

Flora: Perennial, with white and pink flowers May–September.

Folklore: The generic name comes from the classical legend that the Greek hero Achilles used to make poultices from its leaves to treat his warriors after a battle. It has been traditionally used to heal open wounds and stop the flow of blood, hence its popular name of woundwort. In Scandinavian countries it was sometimes used as a substitute for hops. In folklore, yarrow stems featured in divination: young women sewed an ounce of it into a sachet and, placing it under their pillows at night, said,

> Thou pretty herb of the Venus tree,
> Thy true name is Yarrow.
> Who is my true bosom friend to be?
> Pray tell me tomorrow.

They then allegedly went to sleep and dreamed of their future lover. The yarrow used in this love charm had to be picked from a graveyard on the night of the full moon. Yarrow leaves were often hung above the cradles of new-born babies in country districts to protect them from the spells of witches.

General medical properties: Diuretic, antiseptic, digestive, antibacterial and anti-inflammatory.

Specific properties: Medical tests have shown that yarrow stimulates the gastric juices and is therefore an aid to digestion. It also has proven antiseptic and antibacterial qualities and is capable of reducing inflammation.

Application and use: Infuse 1 teaspoon in 1 cup of boiling water for 15 minutes. Take 1 cup a day.

Bibliography

Addey, S. Oddall, *Household Tales*, David Nutt, 1895.

Agrippa, Henry Cornelius, *The Philisophy of Natural Magic*, Antwerp, 1533.

Baker, Margaret, *Discovering the Folklore of Plants*, Shire, 1969.

Ballow, M., *County Folklore: Northumberland*, David Nutt, 1904.

Black, William George, *Folk Medicine*, Elliot Stock, 1893.

Briggs, Katherine M., *The Folklore of the Cotswolds*, Batsford, 1974.

Briggs, Katherine M., *Botonologia: The British Physician or the Nature and Virtue of English Plants*, 1687.

Brown, Theo, 'Charming in Devon', *Folklore*, Vol. 181, spring 1970.

Burnby, J.G.L., *A Study of the English Apothecary 1660–1760*, Wellcome Institute, 1983.

Burne, Charlotte Sophia, *Shropshire Folkore*, Trübner & Co., 1893.

Bryan, Cyril P., *The Ebers Papyrus*, Geoffrey Bles, 1936.

Camp, John, *Magic, Myth and Medicine*, Priory Press, 1973.

Chamberlain, Mary, *Old Wives' Tales*, Virago Press, 1981.

Clark A. *The Working Life of Women in the Seventeenth Century*, Routledge, 1919.

Cockayne, Rev. O., *Leechdoms, Wort Cunning and Star Craft of Early England*, Vols. I and II, Longmans, 1864.

Coles, William, *The Art of Simpling*, 1656.

Creighton, A., *A History of Epidemics*, Cambridge University Press, 1891.

Crow, Dr. W.B., *The Occult Properties of Herbs*, Aquarian Press, 1969.

Cullum, Elizabeth, A Cottage Herbal, David and Charles, 1975.

Culpeper, Nicholas, *Herbal*.

Dawson, W.R., *A Leech Book of Medical Recipes of the Fifteenth Century*, Macmillan, 1934.

Deare, Tony and Shaw, Tony, *The Folklore of Cornwall*, Batsford, 1975.

Drewitt, F. Dawtrey, *The Romance of the Apothecaries Garden at Chelsea*, Chapman and Dodd, 1924.

Ehrenreich, Barbara and English, Deidre, *Witches, Midwives and Nurses*, The Feminist Press, USA, 1973.

Falkland, Richard, *Plant Lore, Legends and Lyrics* Sampson, Masterton & Co., 1892.

'Some Notes on the Pharmacology and Therapeutic Value of Folk Medicines', *Folklore*, Vol. LIX, September and December 1948.

Forbes, T.R., *The Midwife and the Witch*, Yale University Press, USA, 1966.

Friend, Rev. H., *Flowers and Flower Lore*, Vol. II George Allen n.d.

Fulder, Stephen, *The Handbook of Complementary Medicine*, Cornet Books, 1984.

Garland, Sarah, *The Herb and Spice Book*, Frances Lincoln, 1979.

Garrison, Lt. Col., *An Introduction to the History of Medicine*, W.B. Sanders & Co., 1929.

Glyde, John, *The Norfolk Garland*, Jarrold, 1872.

Golsing, Narda, *Successful Herbal Remedies*, Thorson's, 1985.

Gurdon, Lady, *County Folklore: Suffolk*, David Nutt, 1893.

Harner, Michael J., *Hallucinogens and Shamanism*, OUP Inc., USA, 1973.

Hartmann, Dr Franz, *Occult Science in Medicine*, Theosophical Publishing House, 1893.

Henderson, William, *Notes on the Folklore of the Northern Counties of England and the Borders*, W. Satchell, Peyton & Co., 1879.

Hoffman, Dr David, *The Holistic Herbal*, Findhorn/Thorson's, 1984.

Hoffman, Dr. David, *Welsh Herbal Medicine*, Abercastle, 1978.

Hopper, M.M., *Notes on Herbs*, Stoke Lacey Herb Farm, n.d.

Hunt, R. *Popular Romances of the West of England*, 1897.

Huson, Paul, *Mastering Herbalism*, Abacus, 1977.

Inglis, Brian, *A History of Medicine*, Weidenfeld and Nicolson, n.d.

Jones Baker, Doris, *The Folklore of Herefordshire*, Batsford, 1977.

Kloss, Jethro, *Back to Eden*, Back to Eden Books, USA, 1946.

Kremens, E. and Urdang, G., *History of Pharmacy*, J.P. Lippincott, USA, 1944.

Laing, J.M., *Notes on Superstition and Folklore*, John Menzies, 1885.

Law, Desmond, *The Concise Herbal Encyclopedia*, J. Bartholomew, 1973.

Leather, E.M., *The Folklore of Herefordshire*, Sidgwick and Jackson, 1912.

Lehane, Brendan, *The Power of Plants*, John Murray, 1977.

Le Strange, Richard, *A History of Herbal Plants*, Angus and Robertson, 1977.

Lloyd, Gwynedd, *Lotions and Potions*, National Federation of Women's Institutes, n.d.

Lucas, Dr R., *Nature's Medicines*, Award Books, USA, 1968.

Lust, John, *The Herb Book*, Bantam, USA, 1974.

Maple, Eric, *Magic, Medicine and Quackery*, Robert Hale, 1968.

Maple, Eric, 'Witchcraft and Magic in the Rochford Hundred', *Folklore*, Vol. 76, autumn 1965.

Marshall, Simpkin, *The Folklore of East Yorkshire*, Hamilton Kent, 1890.

Miller, P.S.A., *The Magical and Ritual Use of Herbs*, Destiny Books, USA, 1983.

Milton F.V., *Milton's Practical Modern Herbal*, Foulsham & Co., 1976.

Murray, Dr M.A. *The Witch Cult in Western Europe*, Oxford University Press, 1921.

Palaiseul, Jean, *Grandmother's Secrets*, Barrie and Jenkins, 1972.

Peacock, Mabel and Gutch, Mrs, 'Examples of Printed Folklore Concerning Lincolnshire', *County Folklore*, Vol. V, David Nutt, 1908.

Porter, Enid, *The Folklore of East Anglia*, Batsford, 1974.

Porter, Enid, *Cambridgeshire Customs and Folklore*, Routledge, 1969.

Raven, Jan, *The Folklore of Staffordshire*, Batsford, 1978.

Ristater, Carol Ann, *A Dictionary of Medical Folklore*, Thomas Y. Crowell, USA, 1979.

Rivers, Dr W.H.R., *Medicine, Magic and Religion*, Kegan Paul, Trench & Trübner Co. Ltd., 1924.

Robbins, Prof. H., *The Encyclopedia of Witchcraft and Demonology*, Hamlyn, 1970.

Rohde, Sinclair, *The Old English Herbals*, Longman, Green & Co., 1929.

Simpson, Jacqueline, *The Folklore of Sussex*, Batsford, 1973.

Simpson, N.D., A Bibliographical Index of British Flora, privately printed, 1960.

Stabbart, Tom, *Herbs, Spices and Flavourings*, David and Charles, 1970.

Step, Edward, *Herbs and Healing*, Hutchinson, 1926.

Stuart, Malcolm, *The Encyclopedia of Herbs and Herbalism*, Orbis, 1979.

Swinger, Dr Charles, *Early English Medicine and Magic*, Oxford University Press, 1920.

Thiselton Dyer, T.F., *The Folklore of Plants*, Chatto and Windus, 1889.

Thomas, Keith, *Religion and the Decline of Magic*, Weidenfeld and Nicolson, 1971.

Thompson, J.S., *The Mystery and Art of the Apothecary*, Bodley Head, 1929.

Prof. Lynn Thorndike, *A History of Magic and Experimental Science*, Columbia University Press, USA, 1923–58.

Thorne-Quelch, Mary, *Herbs and How To Know Them*, Faber, 1936.

Turner, William, *The New Herball*, 1551.

Tynan, Katherine and Maitland, Frances, *The Book of Flowers*, Smith, Eder & Co. 1909.

Ulydent, Mollie, *The Psychic Garden*, Thorson's, 1980.

Waring, Phillip, *A Dictionery of Omens and Superstitions*, Souvenir Press, 1978.

Weiner, Dr Michael, *Weiner's Herbal*, Stein and Day, USA, 1980.

Whitlock, Ralph, *The Folklore of Wiltshire*, Batsford, 1976.

Woodville, William and Jackson, Dr William, *Medical Botany*, John Bohn, 1932.

Zilboorg, Dr Gregory, *The Medical Man and the Witch in the Renaissance*, Johns Hopkins University Press, USA, 1935.

A SELECTED LIST OF TITLES AVAILABLE IN SENATE

☐	Aborigine Myths & Legends	ISBN 0 09 185039 8	£1.99
☐	Ancient Man in Britain	ISBN 1 85958 207 9	£1.99
☐	The Buddha & His Religion	ISBN 1 85170 540 6	£2.99
☐	Calendars & Constellations of the Ancient World	ISBN 1 85958 488 8	£1.99
☐	Celtic Britain	ISBN 1 85958 203 6	£1.99
☐	Epigrams of Oscar Wilde	ISBN 1 85958 516 7	£2.99
☐	The Folklore Calendar	ISBN 1 85958 040 8	£1.99
☐	Handbook of Folklore	ISBN 1 85958 157 9	£1.99
☐	History & Lore of Freaks	ISBN 1 85958 485 3	£1.99
☐	History of Dreams	ISBN 1 85958 168 4	£1.99
☐	Gestapo	ISBN 1 85170 545 7	£2.99
☐	Immortality	ISBN 1 85958 487 X	£1.99
☐	Lore of the Unicorn	ISBN 1 85958 489 6	£1.99
☐	Mysteries of Britain	ISBN 1 85958 057 2	£1.99
☐	Mythology of the Celtic People	ISBN 0 09 185043 6	£2.99
☐	Phallic Worship	ISBN 1 85958 195 1	£1.99
☐	Who's Who in Shakespeare	ISBN 0 09 185144 0	£2.99

ALL SENATE BOOKS ARE AVAILABLE MAIL ORDER IN THE UK

Please send cheque, postal order, Access, Visa or Mastercard (NOT CASH):

☐☐☐☐☐☐☐☐☐☐☐☐☐☐☐☐ CARD NUMBER

Expiry Date: .... Signature: ....

Total amount of order including p&p: £ .... (INSERT AMOUNT)

UK POST & PACKING:
Allow £2.00 each for first two books and £1.00 each for any books thereafter

ALL ORDERS TO:
Grantham Book Services, Alma Park Industrial Estate, Issac Newton Way,
Grantham, Lincolnshire, NG31 9SD, England
Tel: (01476) 567421   Fax: (01476) 567314

NAME: _____

ADDRESS: _____

_____

Please allow 28 days for delivery
Prices and availability subject to change without notice